FAT DOES NOT MAKE YOU FAT

LATCHMAN HARDOWAR, MD

Dedicate this Book to:

My Parents, wife, Roshnie

daughter, Aaradhya and to my Patients

CONTENTS

INTRODUCTION

One of the most significant things that you need to do in your life for your health as you age is to maintain a healthy weight. It does not matter that you have spent your whole youth in a good shape, but if you are adding pounds in your late 40s or due to any illness, it can be very dangerous for your overall health. Both being underweight and overweight pose challenges for your health.

So if you have been ignoring your weight throughout your life, now is the time that you should give your attention to this aspect of your life. Maintain a healthy weight and get yourself protected from many diseases, such as cardiovascular diseases, poor muscles and bone health, joint pain, etc.

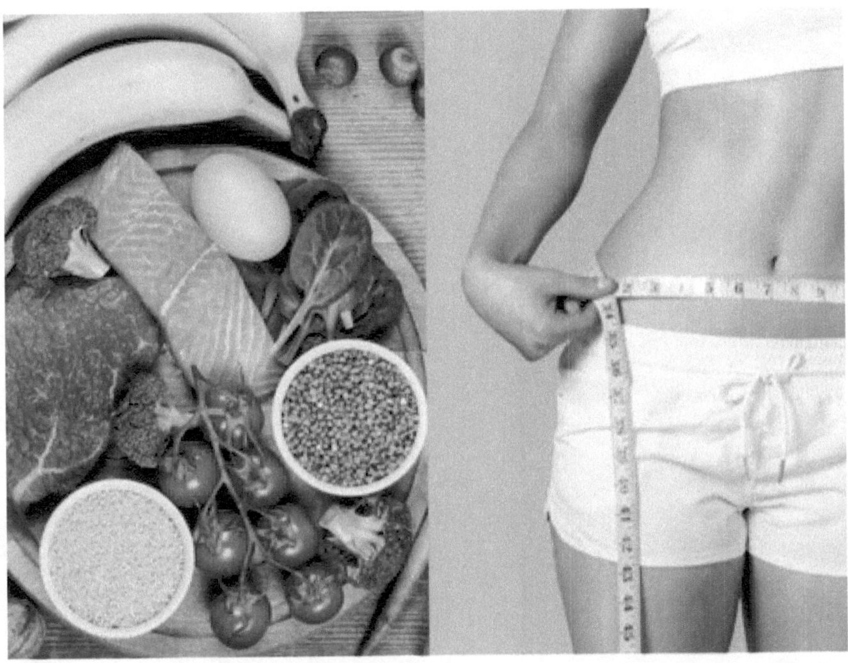

This ebook emphasis on the most easiest and healthy way to lose weight that is having a low carb diet. This ebook unfolds the reasons to go for keto diet along with intermittent fasting, as both together can do wonders to maintain your weight.

01: DANGER OF OBESITY FOR YOUR HEALTH AND HOW TO REVERSE THESE DISEASES?

You are obese when your body has more fat then it is desirable. Obesity has so many harmful effects for your body. If you are suffering from severe obesity, then chances to get different diseases become very high. Some of the most common diseases include sleep apnea, high blood pressure and type 2 diabetes. When these diseases are combined with obesity, it may lead to poor health, ultimately resulting in early death or life time disability. Here are some of the dangers of obesity that shows how it impacts your health.

● Diabetes

Type 2 diabetes is a common chronic illness, cause due to obesity. According to studies, you are ten times more likely to get diabetes if you are obese. Not only this, Type 2 diabetes increases the chances of early death, as well as lead to impotence, infections that are hard to heal, nerve and circulatory defects, hypertension, chronic kidney illness, blindness, stroke, heart diseases and amputations.

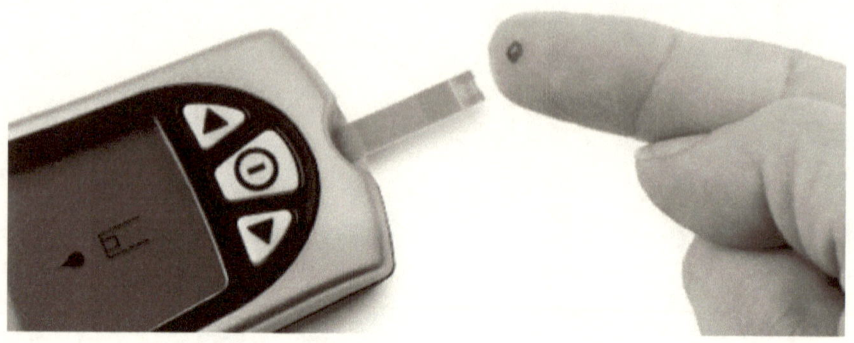

● Hypertension

One of the major reasons that obesity is dangerous for you is it increases the risk for hypertension, also known as high blood pressure. Every 3 out of 4 hypertension cases are because of obesity. Not only this, high blood pressure may lead to diseases, such as CHF (congestive heart failure), CHD (coronary heart disease) and kidney problems.

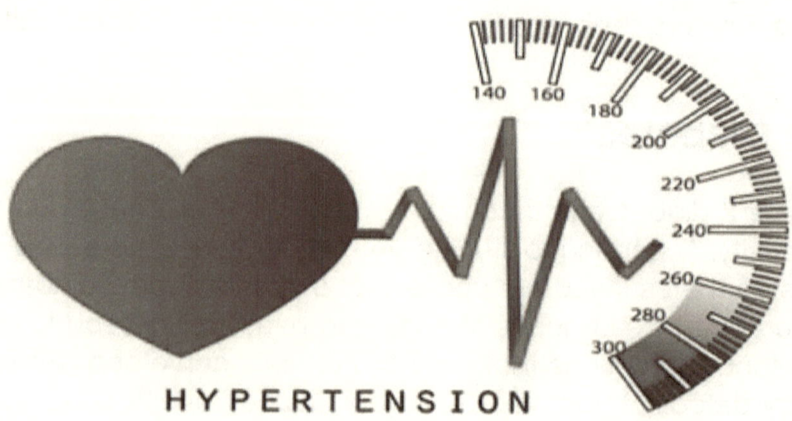

● Heart Disease

In the United States, around 600,000 people die every year because of heart diseases. Obesity is considered as the major reason behind heart diseases as per the American Heart Association. There are several studies that show obesity increases the risk for heart problems. If you are severely obese, you are at a higher risk for heart attack, coronary artery disease and heart failure. In addition, obesity is linked with arrhythmias (irregular heartbeats), which triple the chances of cardiac arrest.

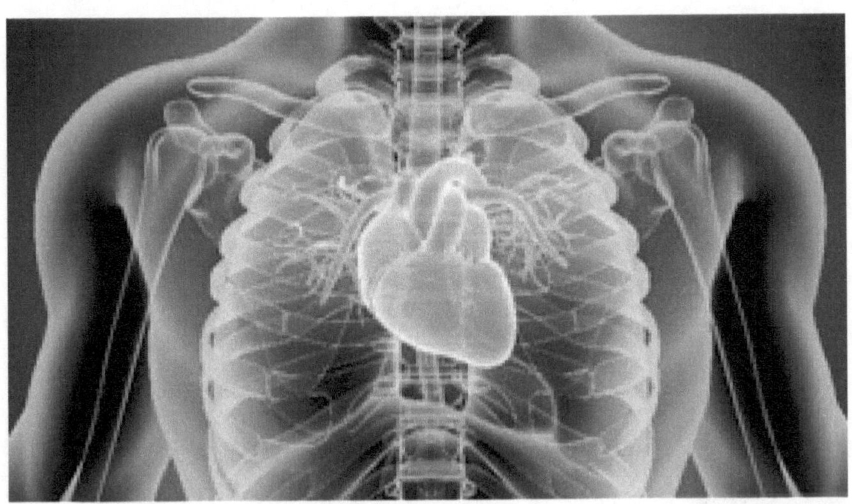

● Respiratory Disorders

The risk for respiratory infections increase when you are obese. You are more likely to get different respiratory disorders, such as asthma. According to studies, asthma is more common among obese people. It has been observed 50 to 60 % people suffering with obesity have OSA (obstructive sleep apnea). The figure increases to 90% in case of severe obesity.

When excess fat in the tongue, throat and neck block air passageways during sleep, OSA occurs. It is a well-known breathing disorder. When there is a blockage, the person is not able to breathe for a time. Each night, a person suffering from OSA has multiple apnea episodes. The amount of oxygen reduces in the person's blood because of apnea episodes. Not only this, OSA also results in heart failure, pulmonary hypertension (high blood pressure), stroke and sudden cardiac death.

This disease affects your sleep in a way that you are not able to get restful sleep as it interrupts your normal sleep cycle, resulting in drowsiness and fatigue.

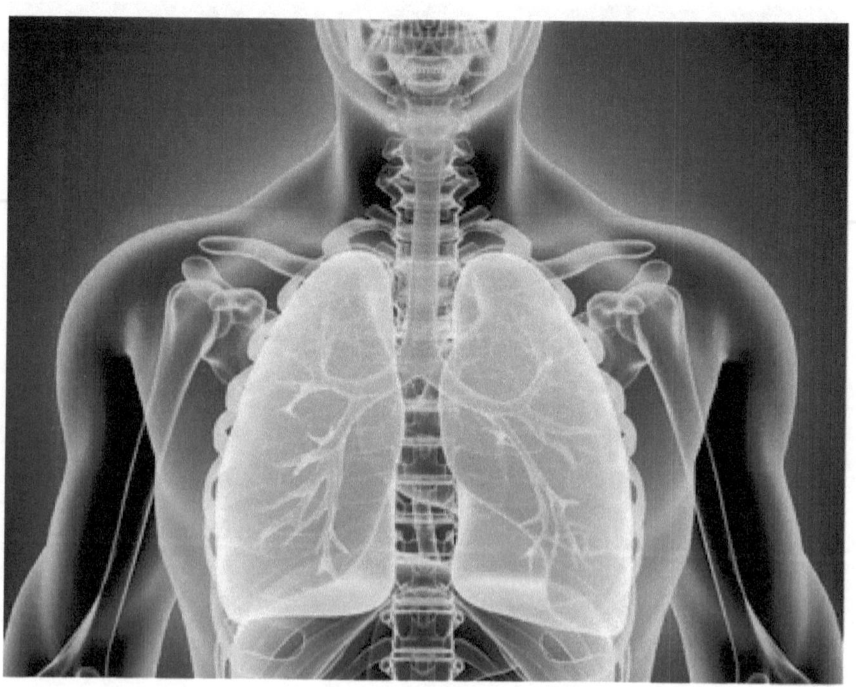

CANCER

In the United States, more than half a million lives are affected due to Cancer every year. It is believed up to 90,000 deaths occur because of cancer resulting from obesity. Your risk of cancer increases as BMI (body mass index) increases. Some of the major cancers include

- Leukemia
- Multiple myeloma
- Non-Hodgkin's lymphoma
- Prostate cancer
- Thyroid cancer
- Kidney cancer
- Liver cancer
- Gallbladder cancer
- Pancreatic cancer
- Esophageal cancer
- Colorectal cancer
- Postmenopausal breast cancer
- Ovarian cancer
- Endometrial cancer
- Cervical cancer

For all types of cancers, the death rate increases for people with severe obesity.

● Cerebrovascular Disease & Stroke

Obesity over-stresses your overall circulatory system and this stress enhances the risk of stroke in your body. Obesity gives rise to other factors as well that lead to stroke. These risk factors include metabolic syndrome, heart diseases, abnormal lipid profile, obstructive sleep disorder, hypertension and type 2 diabetes.

● Gastroesophageal Reflux Disease (GERD)

The health condition called Gastroesophageal Reflux Disease (GERD) results in the leakage of intestinal secretions or stomach acids into your esophagus. Some of the familiar symptoms of GERD are indigestion, heart-burn, vomiting, coughing mostly during night, burping frequently and hoarseness. Around ten percent to twenty percent of people in the world experience these symptoms on a regular basis.

Obesity has mostly been considered as one of the leading causes for GERD and erosive esophagitis, and at times it is also linked with esophageal cancer.

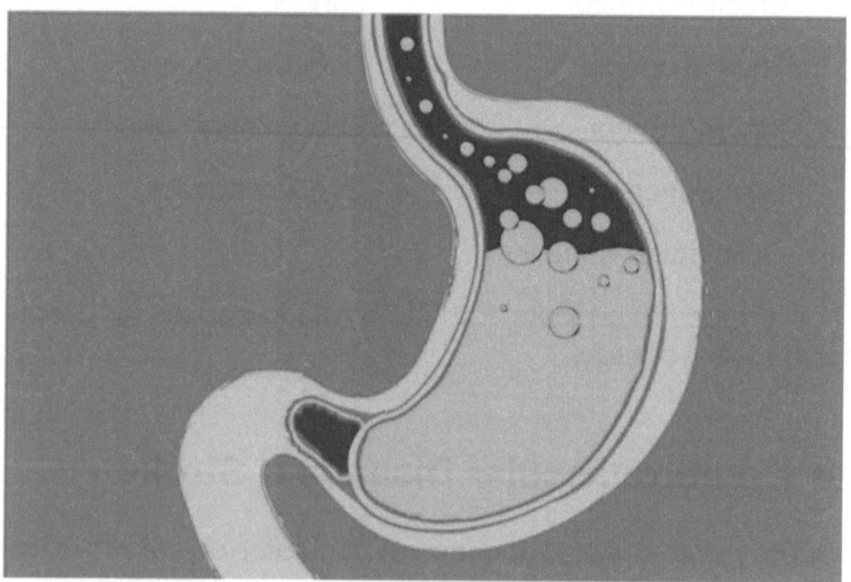

● Damages in Bones/Joints and Accidents

Obesity, particularly severe obesity, leads to numerous problems in your bones and joints. These problems elevate the risks for any serious mishap that can give you a life-time injury. Few of the bone and joint issues are as follows:

- Joint diseases like osteoarthritis

- Spinal disorders

- Disc herniation

- Pseudotumor cerebri, which is a health condition linked with headache, visual impairment and disorientation

- Back pain

OTHER CONDITIONS

- **ALZHEIMER'S DISEASE:** Different medical researchers have concluded that middle-aged obesity patients, when grow older, are exposed to higher risk of health conditions like Alzheimer's disease and dementia.

- **KIDNEY DISEASE:** Type 2 diabetes, cardiac arrest and hypertension are some of the main causes that affect kidney functions and contribute to serious diseases that ultimately lead to kidney failure. All such issues are further worsened by obesity.

- **SEPTICEMIA:** When a severe infection results in a life-taking septic shock, it is called as "septicemia". Medical research has proven that septicemia can catch such people easily who are obese, especially those who are affected by severe obesity.

- **SUICIDE:** Practitioners in the medical field have correlated severe obesity with serious depressive disorder. This means that people with obesity are usually disowned by the society and become prey of discrimination physically and socially. This contributes to depression. Although, strong evidences are not available as whether obesity can be a direct cause of higher suicide rates, but obesity along with other factors causing depression often result in suicidal attempts.

- **LIVER DISEASE:** People who are obese usually suffer from diseases caused by fatty liver and non-alcoholic fatty liver. In fact, severely obese individuals have non-alcoholic fatty liver diseases. Such diseases result in scarring of your liver and weaken your liver functions. If not treated early, you may suffer with cirrhosis and may also experience failure of the liver.

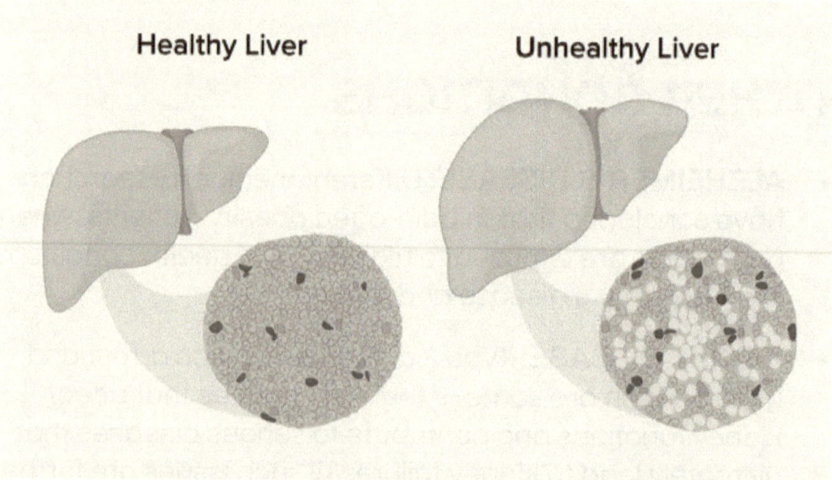

- **FEW OTHER HEALTH CONDITIONS THAT ARE CRITICAL:** These conditions include; preeclampsia and maternal gestational diabetes in pregnant women, higher risks of stillborn and miscarriages, gallbladder infections, pancreatitis etc.

- **DISEASES THAT AFFECT LIFE QUALITY:** These diseases include SUI or stress urinary incontinence, a condition in which urine is leaked out suddenly, skin rashes, infertility, and PCOS or polycystic ovarian syndrome.

HOW TO REVERSE THESE DISEASES?

Obesity impacts your body dramatically. The symptoms of obesity can be harmful to your physical and mental health. However, you can avoid several complications or even some of these can be cured by losing weight.

Since low carb diet promotes weight loss, it is a great treatment for obesity. So if you want to prevent yourself from above mentioned disease, you need to first get rid of obesity, for this follow a low carb diet as well as Intermittent Fasting. First, let's talk about low carb diet.

● What is a Low Carb Diet?

In this fast-paced world where people look for quick weight-loss solutions and effective diet plans, low-carb diets have gained a lot of popularity among health conscious individuals. If you wish to lose pounds in less time period, low-carb diet is definitely a better solution as compared to eliminating carbs completely.

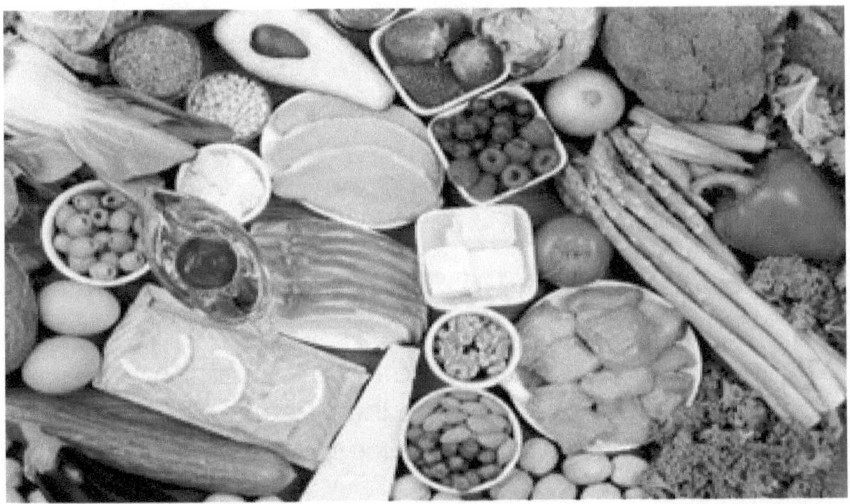

You can define low-carb diet as a dietary routine that allows carbohydrates in a limited amount, including those that you find in starchy vegetables, fruits and grains. You can find a number of low-carb diet plans everywhere, and each of them have some restrictions on intake of carbs on a regular basis.

An example in this regard can be given of "Keto Diet", in which only 5 percent of your overall daily calorie consumption must be from carbohydrates. This concept is completely different from U.S Dietary Guidelines that suggest that forty-five to sixty-five percent of your calorie consumption should be from carbohydrates. Whereas in a 2000-calorie diet plan, 225 to 325 gms of carbohydrate intake is allowed per day.

Undoubtedly, low-carb diet proves highly effective if you wish to lose weight. The low-carb diet not only offers high satisfaction level and major health benefits, but also helps in burning additional calories in your body.

In order to accomplish best results thorough low-carb diet, what you are required to do is:

- Keeping low carbohydrate intake

- Taking protein in moderate amount

- High intake of fat

- Working out regularly

- Avoiding snacking

LOW CARBOHYDRATES, MODERATE PROTEIN, HIGH FAT

When you take the right combination of fat, carbohydrate and protein, you easily lose some pounds. People often get good results with the low-carb diet since most of the heavy carb foods are avoided. These include starchy foods like rice, potatoes, pasta, bread and heavy protein-based foods as well, such as nuts, cheese, and meat.

Many of us do not like monitoring the intake of energy all the time to ensure that we do not cross the limits. However, different types of applications are available in the market which, allow you to measure calorie intake within no time.

● Keeping carbohydrate low

Ketogenic low-carb diets are excellent to achieve weight-loss goals. Carbohydrate intake should be less than 50 grams per day to be a strict ketogenic. With this diet your body is being energized mainly by ketones instead of glucose. When your body fat is broken down to produce energy, ketones are released. To become a ketogenic diet follower, you must cut down starchy foods, some fruits and grains from your diet.

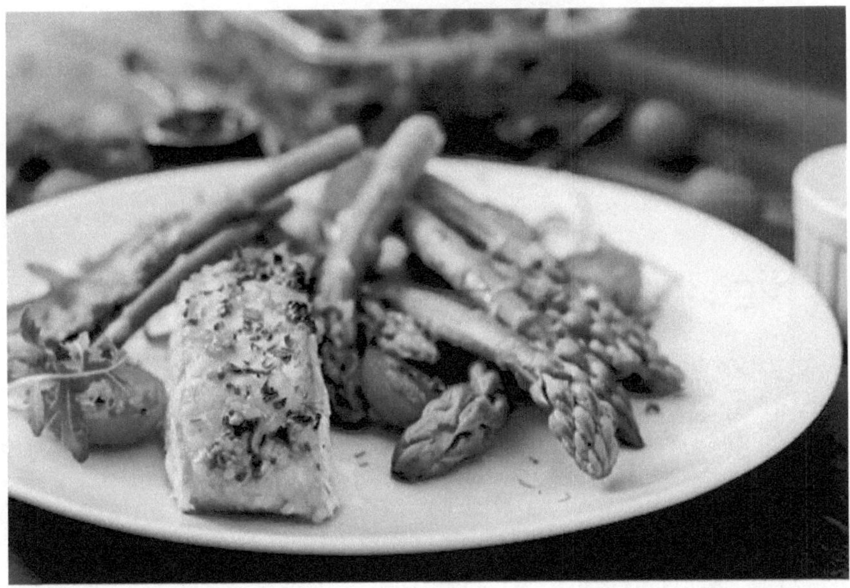

● Protein should be moderate

To lose weight, your protein intake should be moderate. High protein intake leads to high production of glucose by the liver. This raises sugar levels in your body and hence resist weight loss. The term "moderate" does not specify how much protein should be taken but doctors mostly suggest about 30 grams to 120 grams of protein to be consumed. As a beginner, you can start with 50 gm to 60gm of protein per day.

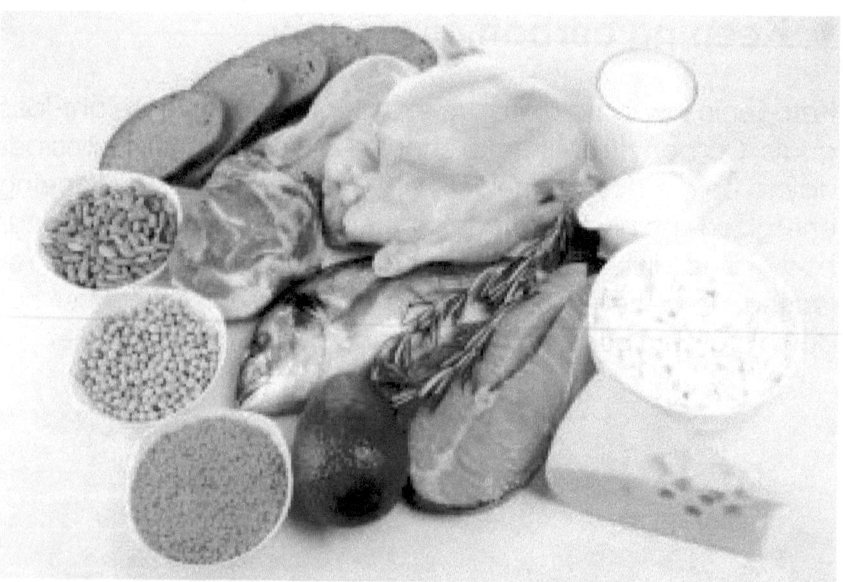

● High in natural fats

A ketogenic diet with low-carb include high fat consumption that may come from organic sources like oily fish, avocado, meats, olive oil, dairy and nuts.

You can define fat as the energy producing nutrient that causes minor effect on insulin levels, blood and weight gain. In other words, a high-fat diet helps tremendously in weight loss compared to diets that include lots of carbohydrates and protein.

One thing that should be kept in mind is that most of the fatty foods like fish, meat, cheese and nuts contain protein, whereas yogurt contain carbohydrates, therefore be careful while consuming high amounts of such foods.

● Avoid snacking

When you follow a low-carb ketogenic diet, you do not find yourself overeating since you stick to a high-fat, moderate-protein, and low-carb diet. You should also remember that no diet gives 100% results and you can achieve weight-loss goals without any difficulty if you omit snacking between your meals. This aids in keeping the insulin level in your body balanced and thus your body burns fat easily.

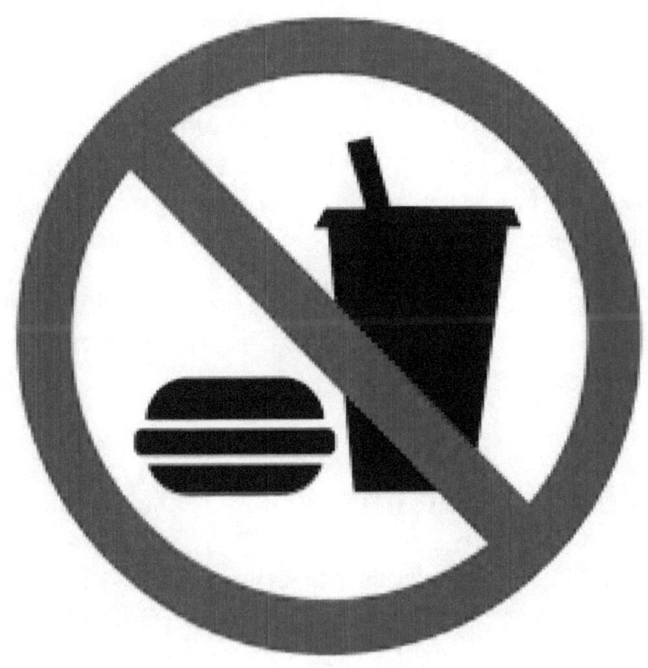

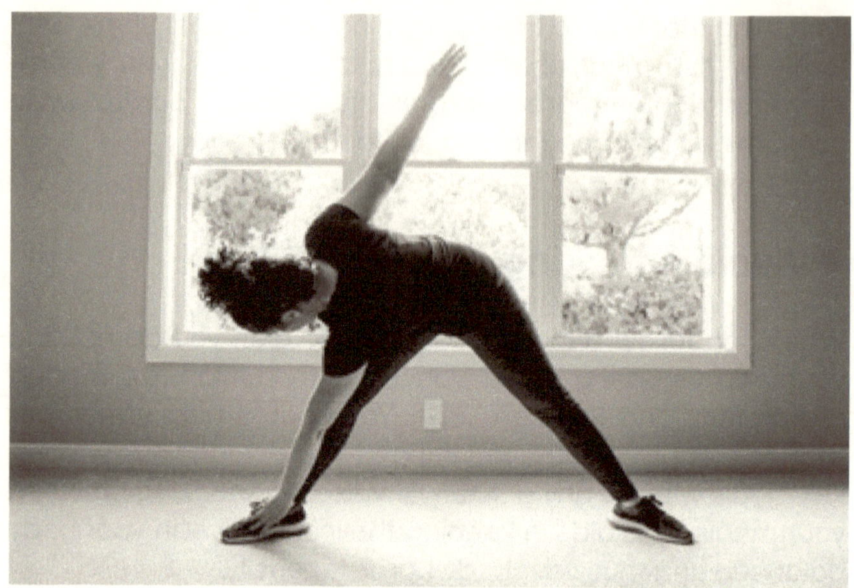

● Exercise regularly

Regular workout keeps your muscles in work and allows them to excrete additional energy and glucose from the blood. This assists in lowering insulin levels, promoting ketosis and stimulating weight loss.

When you make exercise part of your routine along with following a low-carb diet, you also experience a drastic reduction in your waistline.

● Monitor fat burning

Weight-conscious individuals not only measure their weight but also keep a watch on their ketone levels. Since fat burning process results in ketone production, by measuring ketones you can detect whether fat burning in your body is being continued or not.

At times, weight loss may take place because of fluid loss, or you can gain weight by muscle built-up through workout. Hence, ketone measurement aids you in eliminating these uncertainties.

Likewise, ketone measurement is also helpful when you stop losing weight or when you make some changes in your diet. In such cases, you can easily find out if your body is still burning fat or not.

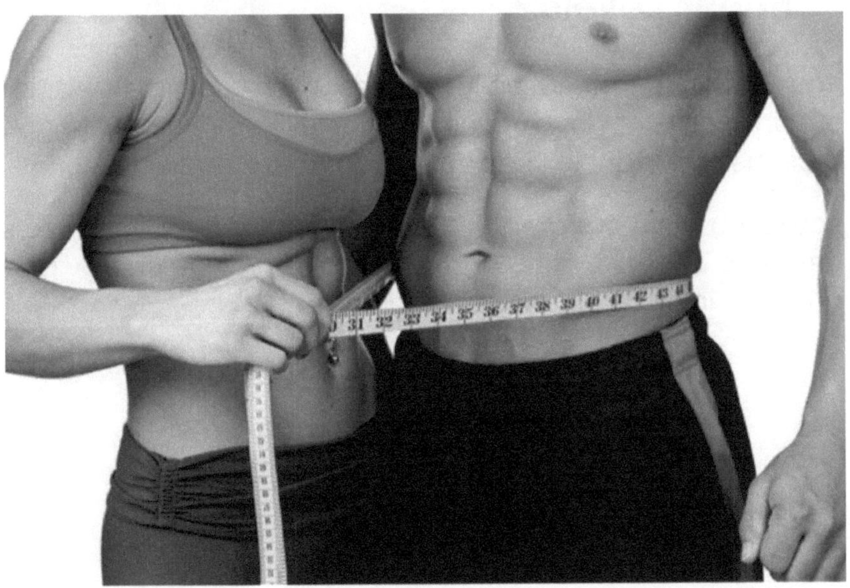

HOW DOES LOW CARB WORK?

You will be happy to read that low carb diets are excellent for people suffering with diabetes. This is because they help in keeping HbA1c levels lower as compared to other diets that creates calorie deficit. Thus, low carb diets promote weight loss. This diet helps in balancing your sugar levels, reduce insulin resistance as well as decrease your appetite between meals. Fat, protein and carbohydrate are the three micronutrients that provide energy, but carbohydrate has the major impact on raising your levels of glucose in the blood, whereas protein has a moderate effect and fat has the least effect. When you take healthy low-carb meals, it becomes easier to maintain your sugar levels as this diet is high in healthy fat, include moderate proteins and very low carbohydrates

● Less Hunger Lead To Steady Sugar Levels

Your appetite automatically reduces when you have steadier sugar levels. Both low and high sugar levels stimulate hunger, thus it is important to keep your sugar at a steadier level.

Low-carb diets are great in keeping you full between meals as intake of healthy fats and vegetables provide energy and nutrients in a sustained and gradual way.

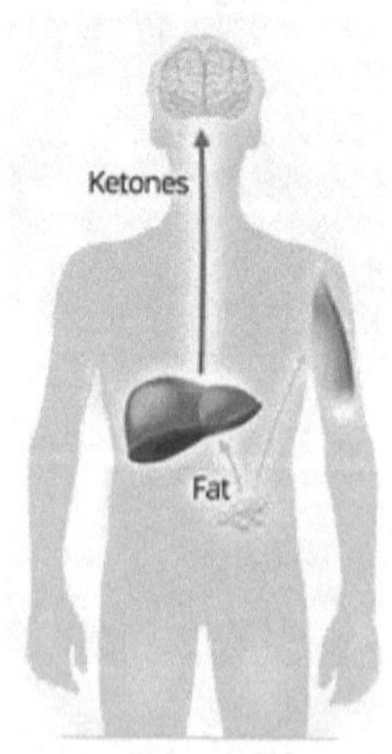

● Ketosis

Ketosis is induced when you take low carb diet that is high in protein and low in carbs. Ketosis is a process when the body starts to break fat and use it as energy. Ketosis is best for people looking to lose weight. There is no specific level of carbs assured to induce ketosis in your body, as there are several other factors well as that are taken into consideration, such as how much exercise you do and protein intake.

The diets that are low in carbs and induce ketosis are known as ketogenic diets. Typically, in a keto diet, you are allowed to take below 50g of carbs daily.

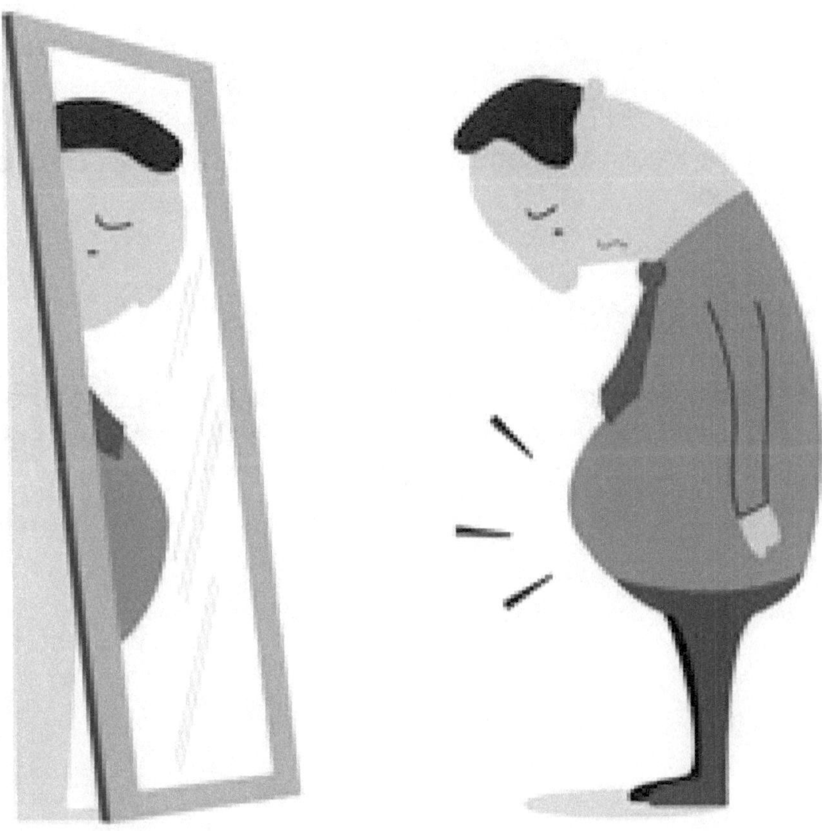

● Reducing Insulin Resistance

Your body releases insulin when you eat just to control the expected increase in blood sugar. Since carbohydrate increases the sugar levels the most, thus carbs require huge amount of insulin released. On the other hand, proteins and fats need smallest insulin release. Here the key player is insulin. This is because when the levels of insulin becomes high, it results in insulin resistance and then ultimately in type 2 diabetes. Therefore, it is essential to decrease insulin resistance in order to improve diabetes and promote weight loss. Reduce the intake of carbs to decrease the amount of insulin in your body and to achieve reduced insulin resistance.

One of the major reasons that people with type 2 diabetes are obese is because their body produces higher levels of insulin and insulin plays an important role in storing body fat. Therefore, insulin is responsible for both insulin resistance and weight gain.

● How To Achieve Weight Loss

Here is a flow chart that shows that how a diet high in carbohydrates initiate events that result in high insulin requirement, high blood sugar and thus weight gain and fat storage.

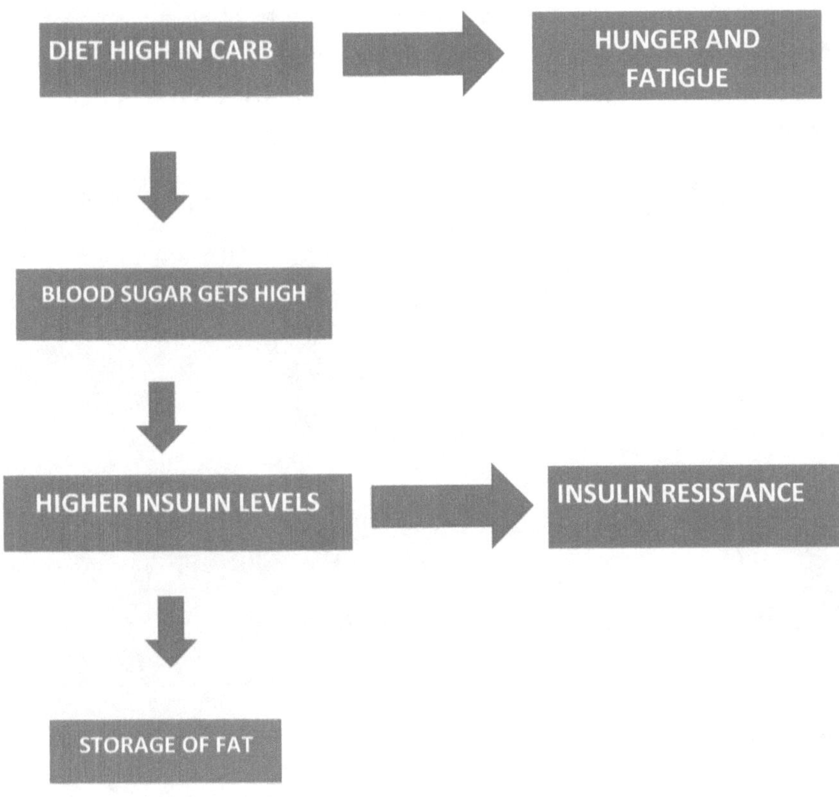

To achieve low levels of insulin, you need to lose weight and here a low-carb diet helps as it is one of the most effective methods of doing this. The low carb diet helps you in maintaining a normal eating schedule, at the same time keeping insulin levels in range and lower storage of fat.

Besides dieting, you also need to keep yourself physically active, as this burns body fat as well as lowers your sugar level.

TIPS TO FOLLOW A LOW CARB DIET

It is an amazing decision to follow a healthy low-carb diet. The diet basically focuses on a variety of mouth-watering vegetable dishes. Since low carb diet is a lifestyle change, therefore it needs to be easier to follow and equally enjoyable. Once you will switch to a low carb diet, you will realize that it is not only healthy but also satisfying for your taste buds.

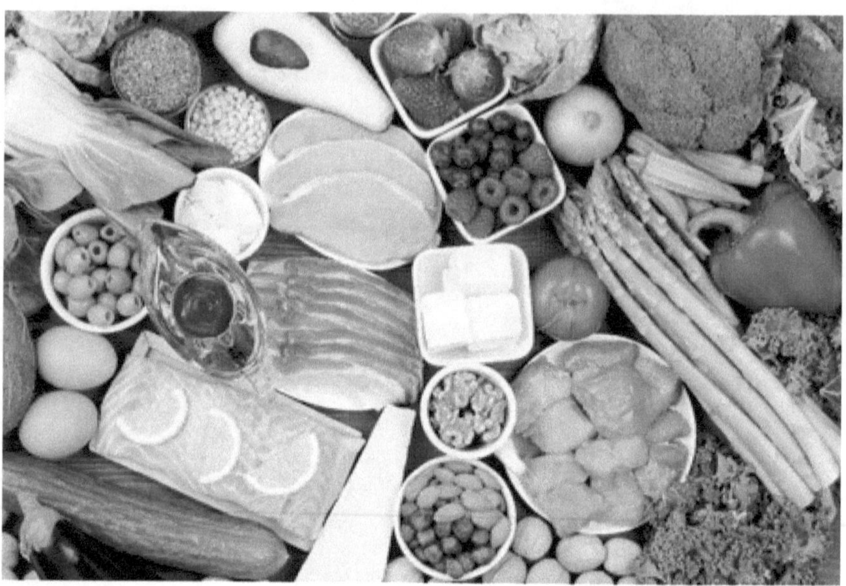

Following are some of the basic points that you need to follow while being on a low carb diet.

- You need to increase the intake of vegetables.

- Have protein in moderate amount

- No or very little processed food.

- Eat less or no fruits

- Have less sugary or starchy foods

- Include natural and healthy sources of fat

- A moderate amount of protein

One of the biggest advantages of following this diet is that there is no involvement of grains, thus it becomes easier to have vegetables in large portions. To make your low carb diet successful, you need to put some effort and time in preparing and cooking the meals. This is the only way you can convert vegetables into truly delicious meals.

● Healthy Fats

When following a low carb diet, you need to take most of your energy from natural sources of fats, such as avocado oil, nut oils, coconut oil, olive oil, coconut based foods, nuts, olives, avocado, dairy, oily fish and meat.

The focus is on fat on a low carb diet because it gradually provides energy that helps in keeping you satisfied for a longer period of time. However, you need to take moderate amount of some healthy fat sources, for example, cheese and nuts, as they also contain a lot of protein.

Make sure to exclude unhealthy fatty foods from your diet as they high in carbohydrate, for example, sausage rolls, fries, chips, crisps and pies.

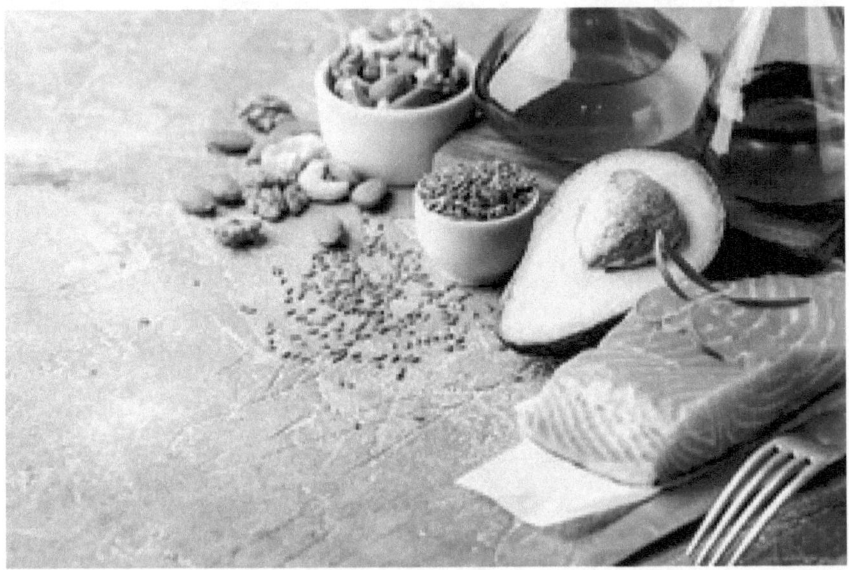

● Protein

There are several sources of protein, including lentils, legumes, nuts, bean, dairy, eggs, meat and fish. Some of these foods, such as nuts are also a good source of fat, while some contain large amount of carbohydrates also, including lentils, legumes and beans.

You need to have very little or no such foods that contain carbohydrates if you are following a ketogenic (low carb) diet.

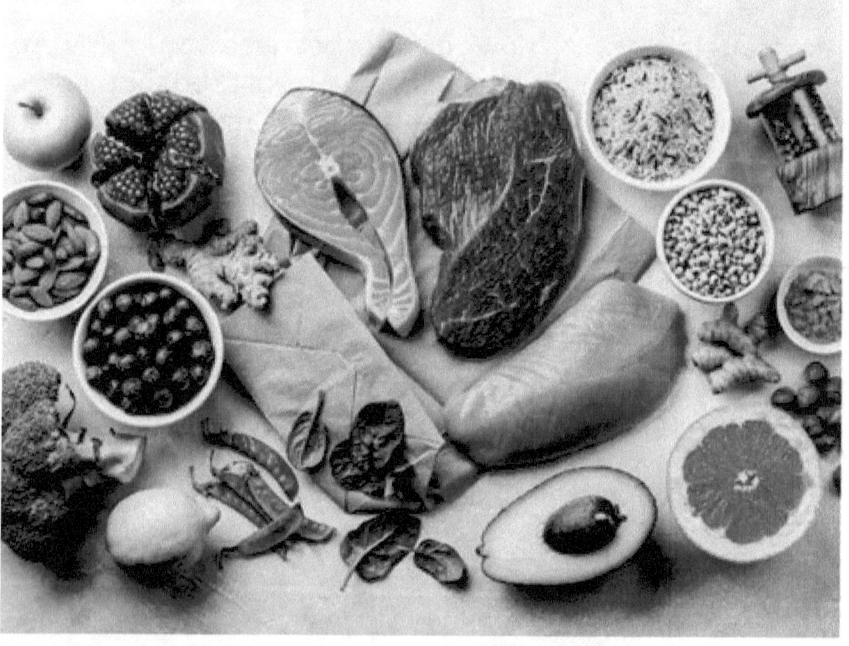

WHAT IS AN INTERMITTENT FASTING AND HOW IT HELPS IN WEIGHT LOSS?

You must have listened about intermittent fasting, but do you actually know what it is and how it impacts your body weight and why it is one of the latest and most popular fitness trend? Your all questions will be answered now! Basically, intermittent fasting involves alternating cycles of eating and fasting.

There are a number of studies that show that Intermittent Fasting helps you to live longer, protect you against diseases, improve metabolic health and cause healthy weight loss.

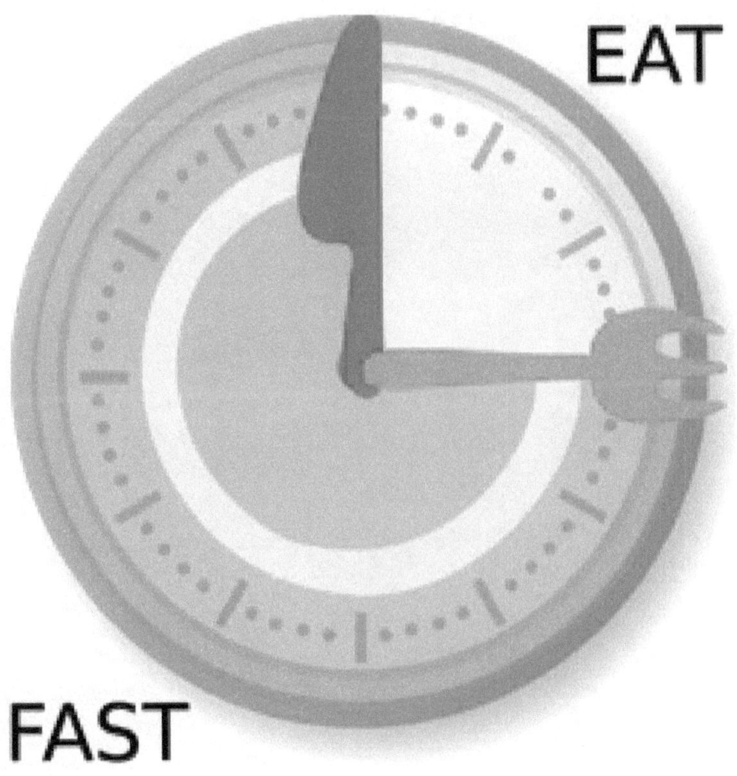

● What Is Intermittent Fasting?

It is a pattern of eating where you give gaps between your cycles of fasting and eating. The science behind this type of fasting is that you do not have to be conscious regarding what you eat, instead you need to take care of when you eat. There are a number of different methods to do intermittent fasting, which splits the week or the day into fasting periods and eating periods.

You can fast simply by skipping your breakfast. Have food at noon and then your final meal at 8 pm. In this way, you are fasting technically for 16 hours daily, while limiting the eating time to an 8-hour period. This method is known as the 16/8 intermittent fasting. You will get to know about intermittent fasting in details in other chapters.

02: CUTTING DOWN CALORIES IS NOT A CURE FOR OBESITY

Every individual likes to keep his/her body in shape. There are numerous ways to keep your body fit physically. One of the prominent ways to acquire a perfect physique or shed few pounds is to cut down calories from your diet.

Now, you can set the target about how many calories you wish to cut down. Then, according to your set target, you can reduce your meal portions or may even skip meals. However, when you touch the extremities of the low-calorie diet, you start experiencing adverse effects of the diet rather than the benefits that could have helped you accomplish balanced weight.

Before heading towards the negative effects of following a low-calorie diet, following are a few points that should be discussed:

CALORIE IS NOT JUST A CALORIE

Obesity is majorly caused when you eat a lot but do not burn it through exercise. It mostly depends on your likings that you love eating too much food but avoid body movement. In fact, you are solely responsible for adding up junk in your body since you choose to have burger or pizza instead of eating nutritious salad. Likewise, you could have spent an hour in the gym instead of playing video games on your PC. Thus, this unhealthy lifestyle exceeds calorie intake over calorie consumption, and you end up gaining weight.

What people assume is that it does not matter what you eat, it is just a calorie and all types of calories are equally likely to gain weight. Basically, a calorie is just a form of energy. When certain foods are burned, this energy is released. Some foods contain less calories while others contain more. In this case, it doesn't matter whether these meals are carbohydrate, fat or protein, it all gets burned in our body and from here we can find out the amount of heat released. And what matter the most is the total daily caloric intake when it comes to gaining weight. So whether you eat ice cream or salad, in the end, it all will be converted into calories.

BUT THE TRUTH IS

Calorie is not just a calorie because when we eat (our dietary habits) and what to eat (specific foods) has a great impact on our metabolic rate. Thus, food behavior and your food choices have the tendency to change TEE (Total Energy Expenditure).

Moreover, it has also been proved through various studies that when you increase the intake of calories, it will also raise the Calories Out and when you decrease the intake of calories, it leads to the deduction in Calories Out. Thus, this likely to change the impact of decrease or increase of calorie intake. All your life, when you thought that eating less is a cure of obesity, here is the reality check. Instead of focusing on the scale of intake and burning up of calories, we should understand that our body acts much more like a thermostat. In simple words, our body has a specific BSW (Body Set Weight). If you make any attempt to raise it above BSW, the TEE will increase (excess calories are burnt due to faster metabolism) and your body will get back to its original weight. In the same way, if you make any attempt to reduce it below BSW, the TEE will decrease (lost calories are regained due to a slower metabolism) and your body will get back to its original weight.

YOU TEND TO EAT MORE IN DIETING!

Have you ever noticed that whenever you go on a diet, you crave to eat more? You feel hungry all the time since the hormones responsible for your hunger, called "ghrelin" increase tremendously whereas satiety hormones decrease. Consequently, you do not feel full and want to eat more. If you go deep into the science of your body then you will find that it has a specific Body Set Weight (BSW). Now, if you assume that your BSW is 250 pounds, you try to cut down calories, however maintain the macronutrient content, like 40% carbohydrates, 30% protein and 30% fat. With these values, you are going to lose weight for a certain time period, maybe till 200 pounds. Since BSW remains the same, that is 250 pounds, your body will try to acquire the same value that is 250 pounds. The immediate reaction is that you raise your calorie intake. Your body does all this by enhancing ghrelin and decreasing satiety hormones. In this way, you feel hungry and fill your stomach. The reduction in weight also lowers the overall energy expenditure, and so your body's metabolism is affected severely and becomes slow.

The aforementioned details highlight that hormones dominate our feelings and make you feel cold, hungry, depressed and exhausted. All these effects are true and measurable results of limiting calories. Therefore, you can conclude that limiting calories causes your body to get back to its real weight as soon as possible. You become hungry and your body's metabolism process is nearly stopped to save calories in order to reach the original weight.

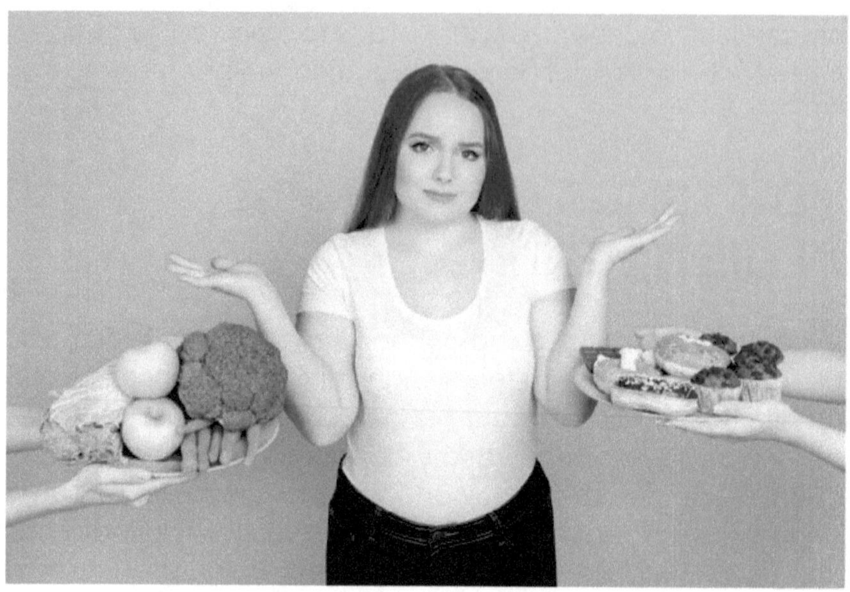

HOW CAN YOU DEFINE CALORIE DEFICIT?

We can define calorie deficit as the energy gap, which occurs due to expansion of more energy than absorption from food within a certain period of time (particularly each day). When this calorie deficit is created, your body is forced to cover for this energy shortfall by using its energy stores.

The energy stores referred here include stored carbohydrates or glycogen, muscle tissues or stored protein and body fats or stored fat. Since glycogen is present in limited amount, the maximum possible energy is dragged from fat cells during weight loss, without affecting the muscle mass of the body.

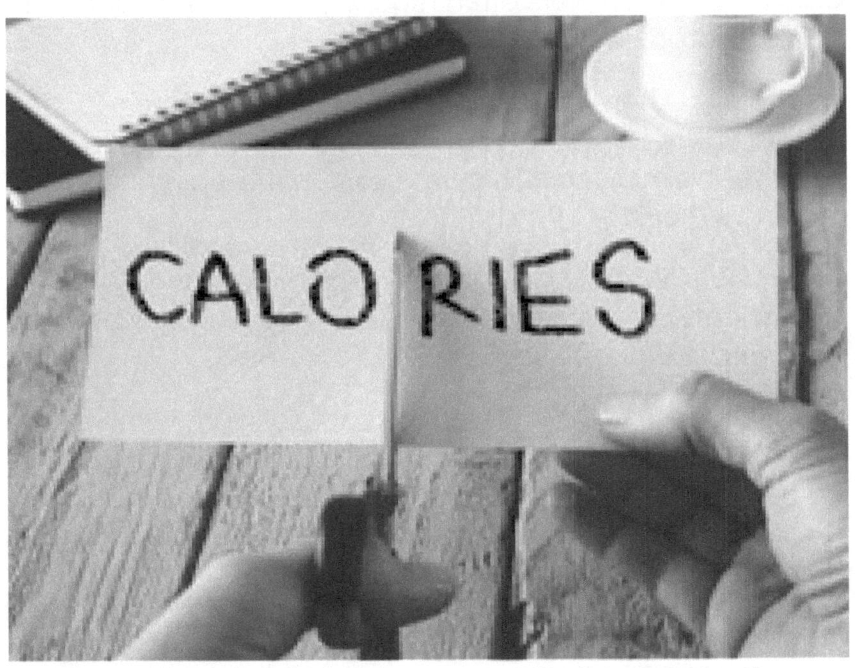

SIDE-EFFECTS OF LOW-CALORIE DIET ON YOUR HEALTH

● Causes Exhaustion and Nutrient Deficiencies

When you take calories less than your body needs, it makes you exhausted, and it becomes difficult for you to cover up with your daily nutrient requirements. For instance, low-calorie diets may cause deficiency of vitamin B12, folate or iron. Consequently, you may become anemic and experience extreme fatigue.

Calorie-restricted diets often require you to limit other essential nutrients as well, like:

- Protein: When you do not eat enough high-protein foods such as meat, dairy, fish, beans, lentils, peas, seeds and nuts, this may result in muscle loss, brittle nails and thinning of hairs.

- Calcium: When your intake of calcium-rich foods is less like leafy greens, dairy, and milk, then your bones become weak and this raises the risk of fractures.

- Thiamine and Biotin: Thiamine and biotin are two important B vitamins that you get from legumes, whole grains, dairy, eggs, seeds and nuts. When you limit the intake of these foods, it causes loss of hair, muscle strength, and results in scaly skin.

- Magnesium: Deficiency of magnesium in your body causes migraines, fatigue, abnormal heart-beat and muscle cramps. By limiting nuts, leafy greens and whole grains you become magnesium deficient.

- Vitamin A: When you do not consume enough vitamin A-rich foods such as fish, leafy greens, dairy, organ meat, or vegetable and fruits, this weakens your immune system and damages your eyes' health.

Hence, to avoid exhaustion and nutrient deficiencies, do not cut down your calories completely and make sure that you include organic or low-processed foods in your diet.

● Nausea

Due to lack of nutrients in your body, especially low sodium and carbohydrates, you may experience a feeling of nausea. When the situation becomes worse, you may even face visual disturbances because of extreme weakness.

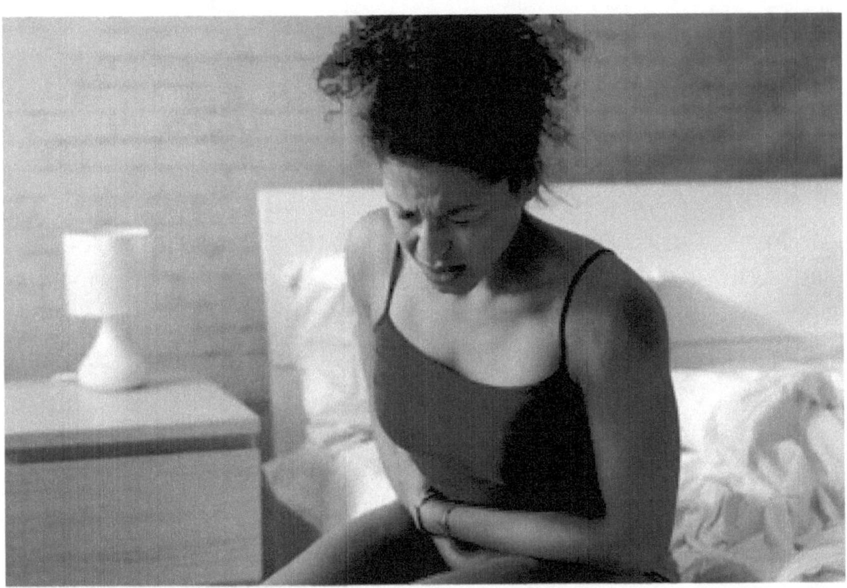

● Headaches

Headaches are another side-effect of losing weight rapidly. Headaches usually occur due to low sugar levels in blood. Drinking plenty of water throughout the day may help but the most important thing is to raise your calories.

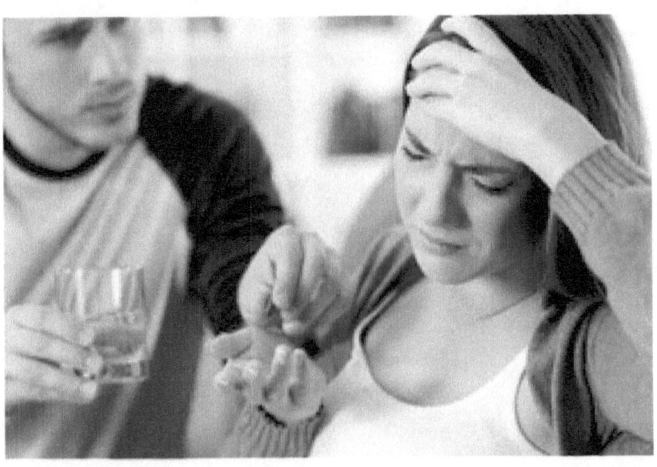

● Constipation

Constipation is a condition when your bowel movements are irregular and have difficulty in passing stool. In this state, you feel uneasy even if you are taking less food.

As low-calorie diets prohibit eating normal quantity of food as well, you end up taking less fiber and carbs and often suffer from severe constipation. Seeking a fiber supplement or consuming any vegetable or fruit with high fiber content can help in such situation.

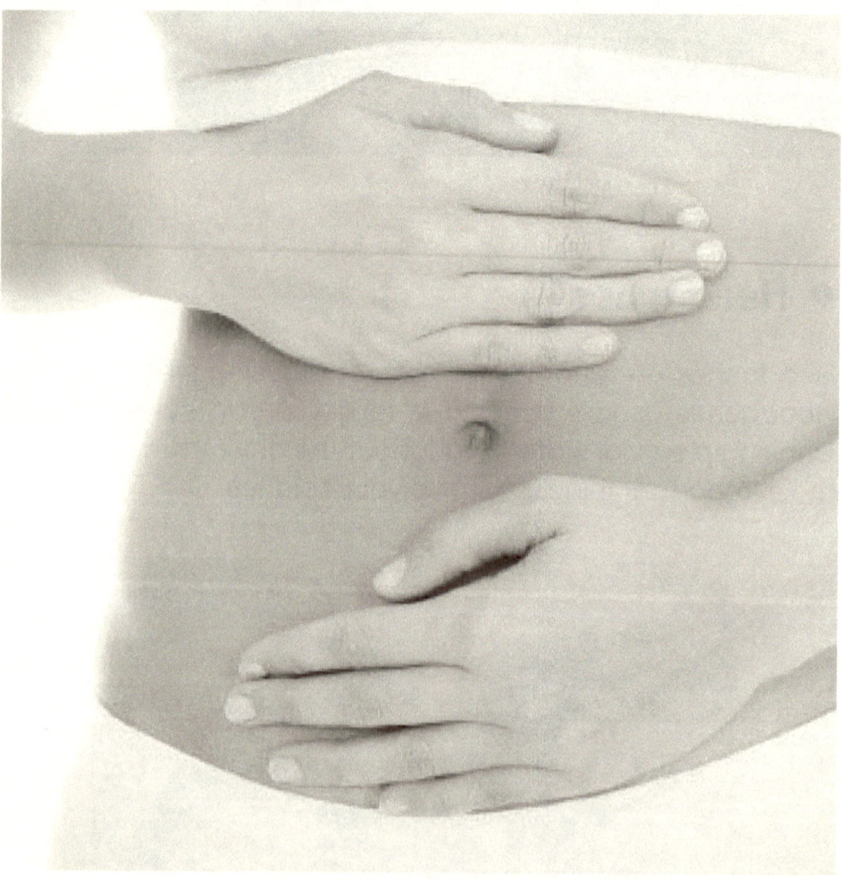

● Gallstones

When you lose a lot of weight within a short span of time by limiting calories, it enhances cholesterol levels in the gallbladder and suppresses its ability of excreting bile. As a result, gallstones are formed. They can be defined as digestive fluid deposited as a hard substance in your gallbladder that causes severe pain, high body temperature and yellowish skin.

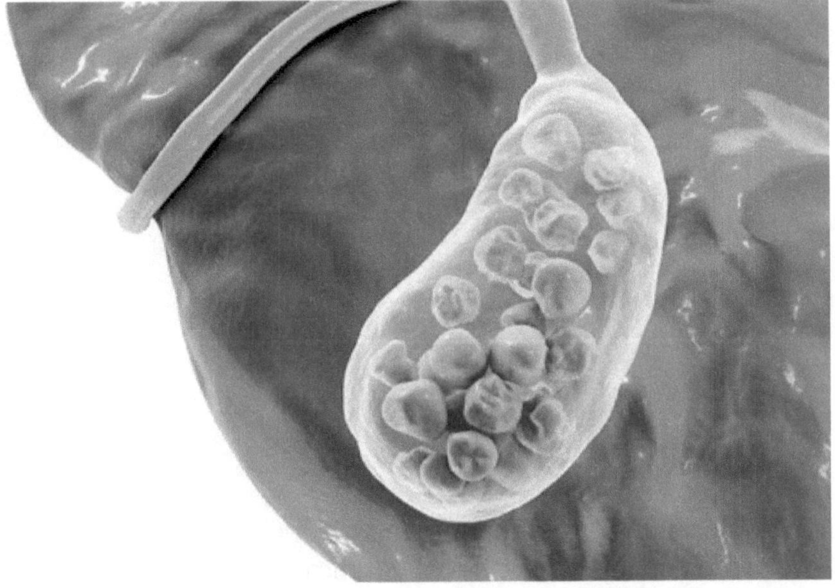

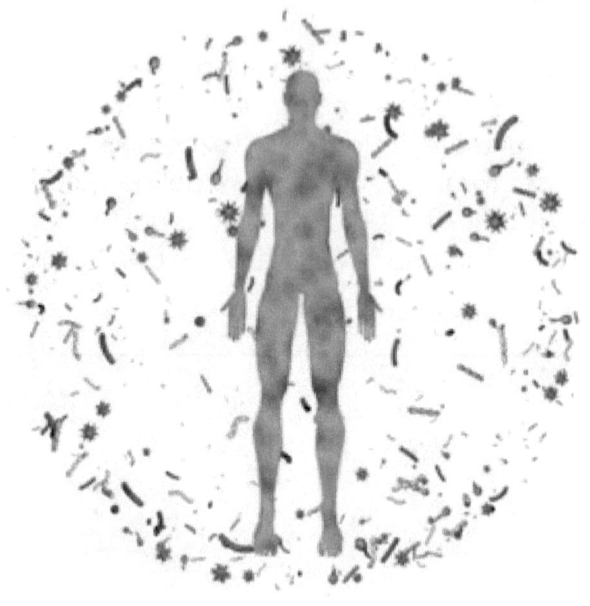

● Immunity

Low-calorie diet restrictions make you iron deficient with low-protein levels. This affects your immune system and your body loses its ability to fight off flu, cold and other severe diseases.

When you increase calorie intake to cope up for energy loss, the adverse effects on the immune system are reversed.

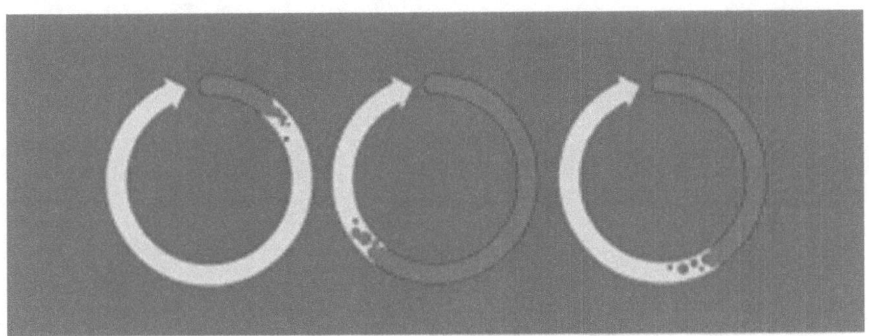

● Pregnancy and Menstruation

Low consumption of calories also disturbs the menstrual cycle in women or may even stop the periods completely. As soon as your periods stop, the risk of bone loss increases because of low estrogen and calcium. This may initiate the process of osteoporosis and can cause broken bones. Similarly, if a pregnant woman takes low-calorie diet, there are chances that the baby experiences delays in growth and development, and may also born with damaged organs.

● Weight Loss and Metabolism

Another crucial side-effect of a low-calorie diet is that your body assumes that it is in starvation mode. This makes it to lose the muscles that boost metabolism rather than fat, thus causing your weight-loss efforts to go in vain.

It also slows down metabolism altogether and causes difficulty in losing weight later.

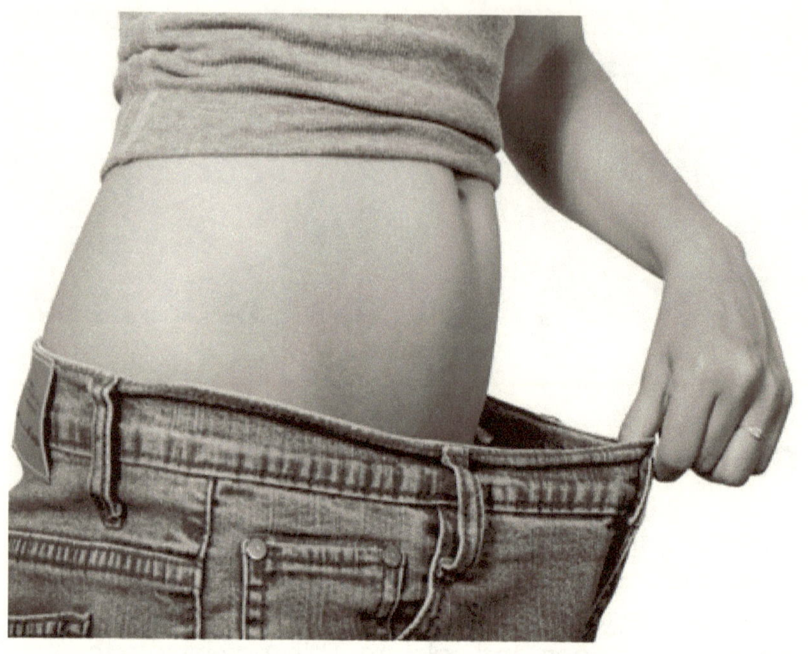

● It Can Make Your Bones Weak

Calorie-restricted diet reduces testosterone and estrogen levels in your body. These reproductive hormones slow down bone formation and enhance bone breakdown, thus making your bones weak.

Similarly, the physical exertion of the body along with low-calorie diet can raise stress hormone levels in your body, consequently causing loss of bones, which is irreversible.

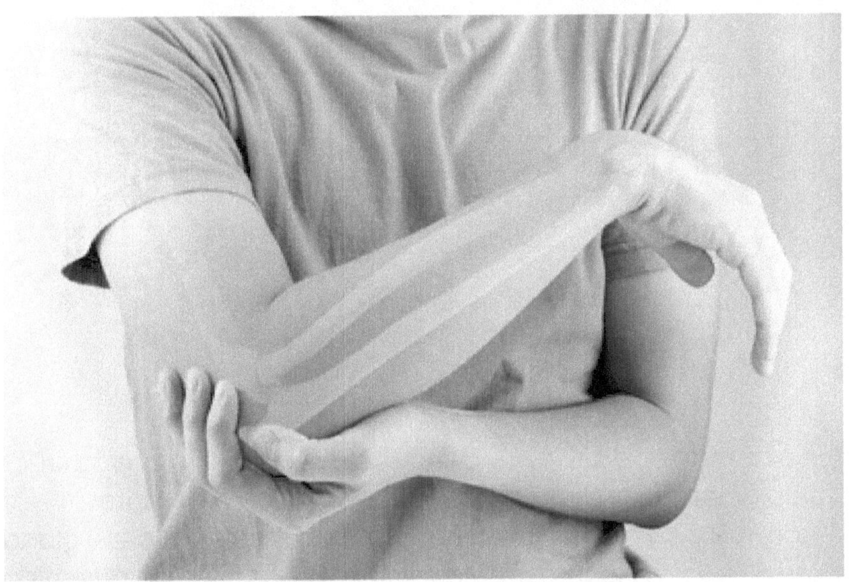

● Other Effects

Other effects of low-calorie diet include:

- low-blood pressure

- issues with heart rhythm

- baldness or loss of hair

- brittle nails

- problems in concentrating

- weak coordination

- muscle weakness, anemia and swelling of joints

03

OVERPRODUCTION OF INSULIN IS THE CAUSE OF OBESITY

In a human body, the pancreas is responsible for the production of insulin. Pancreas is a portion of the small intestine. It acts not only as an exocrine gland, but also endocrine gland as well. As an exocrine gland, the pancreas helps in digesting the food, whereas its endocrine function is to produce insulin and a hormone, known as glucagon.

There are certain beta cells in the pancreas that generate insulin. These cells exist in the form of cluster and are grouped together to be called as islets of Langerhans. You can find around 1 million islets in the pancreas of a healthy individual. The cells in the pancreas that generate glucagon are known as "alpha cells".

WHAT IS THE PURPOSE OF INSULIN IN YOUR BODY?

Insulin is a hormone that stores energy. When you take any meal, it aids the body cells in using carbohydrates, protein and fats whenever the need arises, and also stores the remaining energy, primarily in the form of fats for future consumption. The nutrients are then broken down into molecules of sugar, lipid and amino acids. All such molecules also undergo the process of conversion into highly complex molecules.

● What is Carbohydrate Metabolism?

When you eat food, your sugar levels in blood rises, however carbohydrates play a significant role in the sudden increase in sugar levels. Your digestive system works to convert food into glucose, which is then absorbed in your blood. As the level of glucose rises, the pancreas releases insulin to remove it from your blood. Insulin performs its task by binding with insulin receptors that are present on the body cell surface. It acts as a key that give an opening to the cells to accept glucose molecules. Insulin receptors exist on around all the tissues of the human body.

Insulin receptors mainly consist of two elements—the interior and exterior parts. Now, the exterior part of the receptor connects with insulin by extending outside the cell. When this occurs, the interior portion of the receptor releases a signal within the cell that activates glucose transporters to move towards the cell surface and accept glucose. When levels of sugar and insulin reduce in blood, the glucose transporters move back inside the cell.

If your body functions are normal, the glucose obtained from carbohydrates is removed quickly with the help of this process. However, in case where insulin level is zero or is quite low, the glucose remains in your blood, thus causing high blood sugar levels that stay constant.

You will find excessive blood sugar level in your body when insulin is not used properly by cells. Insulin resistance may occur because of inappropriate insulin shape, due to which receptor binding does not take place. Other reasons for insulin resistance include; less number of insulin receptors, inactive glucose transporters, issues with signaling and excess fat in the body.

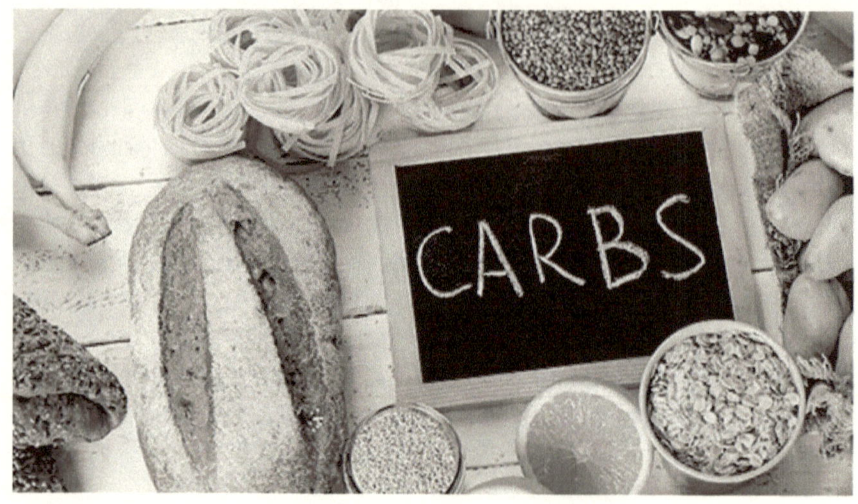

● What is Fat Metabolism?

Your body's fat metabolism is majorly affected by insulin. When you take a meal, the additional glucose and ingested fats are stored by insulin in the form of fat, to be used in the future. Other important roles of insulin include:

The Liver: The production and storage of glycogen using glucose is initiated by insulin. When insulin levels increases, your liver is filled with glycogen and so it prevents further storage. Thereafter, glucose is utilized to produce fatty acids, which later convert into lipoproteins and then into free fatty acids. Other tissues use these free fatty acids for creating triglycerides in your body.

Fat Cells: The existence of insulin in your body prevents the conversion of triglycerides and fat into fatty acids. As glucose become part of these cells, a compound known as glycerol is formed. When glycerol combines with additional free fatty acids, it results in the formation of triglycerides. These triglycerides are then built up into the fat cells in the body.

● What is Protein Metabolism?

The role of insulin also involves making easy entrance of amino acids present in protein, into cells. When insulin is not produced in adequate amount, this process is affected greatly, thus preventing formation of muscle mass.

Your body cells readily accept electrolytes, (which include phosphate, magnesium and potassium) due to the presence of insulin. These electrolytes aid in conducting electricity within your body. During this process, they affect pH of blood, fluid amount in your body and muscle function. High sugar levels in the blood may result in electrolyte imbalance and consequently you may urinate excessively.

HAZARDS OF FRUCTOSE AND SUGAR

● Sugar

Undoubtedly, sugars promote fattening and there is no difference of opinion about this statement. Sugar acts as empty calories in your body, since it consists very little important nutrients. It is a form of carbohydrate and so this is a crucial factor in promoting fattening of body. When you add sugar in any food, it makes its taste pleasant and often causes overeating and ultimately results in obesity.

When we consider the hazards of fructose then we find that although it is not responsible for raising blood sugars significantly, but it has a deep connection with diabetes and obesity as compared to glucose. Fructose is similar to glucose in as sense that it also offers empty calories. Now, the question arises that why it is dangerous to our health?

Before going deep into the topic, we must first understand certain definitions. Glucose is actually a six ringed sugar, which is present in your blood. Almost every cell in the body can utilize glucose. For instance, it acts as a major source of energy in brain. Likewise, muscle cells derive it from the bloodstream for an instant boost of energy. Liver stores glucose in different forms like glycogen. When your body is under stress, glucose is released for boosting energy quickly. In fact, glucose keeps circulating throughout your body without any limitations.

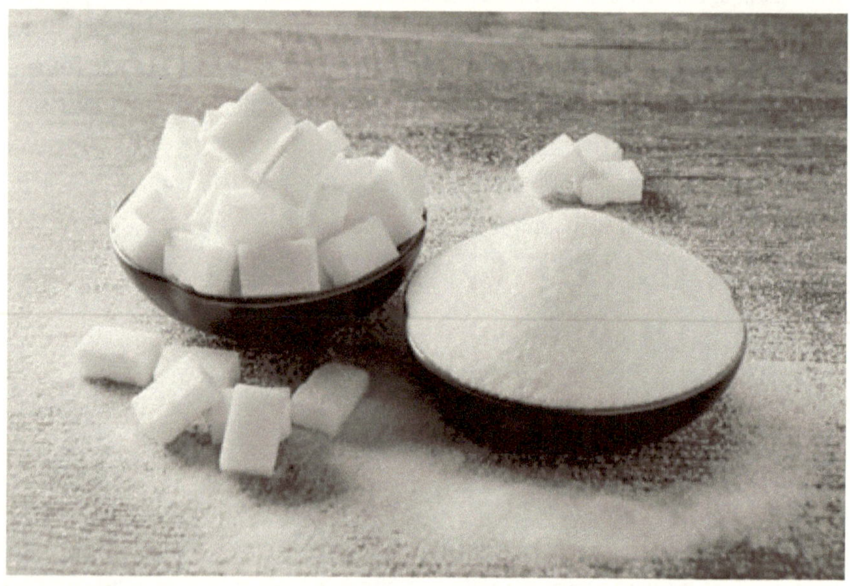

On the contrary, fructose is a five ringed sugar, which is a natural ingredient in fruits. The Liver metabolizes this sugar and it no more circulates as fructose as your body is incapable of using fructose in its original form. For instance, your muscles and brain have no ability to use fructose. That is the reason why, the ingestion of fructose does not considerably alter the sugar levels in blood. The real issue with the sugars like fructose and sucrose is the amount consumed or dosage. Today sugar intake is increasing day by day and this has been closely associated with the increasing diabetes and obesity rates.

● Sugar Sweetened Beverages

Sugar sweetened beverages (SSB) cannot be ignored whenever sugar is discussed. These SSBs include; sodas, soft drinks, sweetened juices and teas etc. For adults as well as children, the intake of juices and SSB has risen tremendously. Diabetes is a disease that occurs due to sugar rather than calories. Type 2 Diabetes arises when extensive amount of sugar is stored in your body, and here we refer to the total body sugar.

The main issue in treating type 2 diabetes is that only blood sugar can be controlled by inducing it in your body mostly in the liver. Such treatments, like insulin, have failed to minimize the complexities created by diabetes. Hence, you can say that insulin is only helpful in treating the blood sugars, and not cures diabetes as it fails to eliminate the sugar from your body.

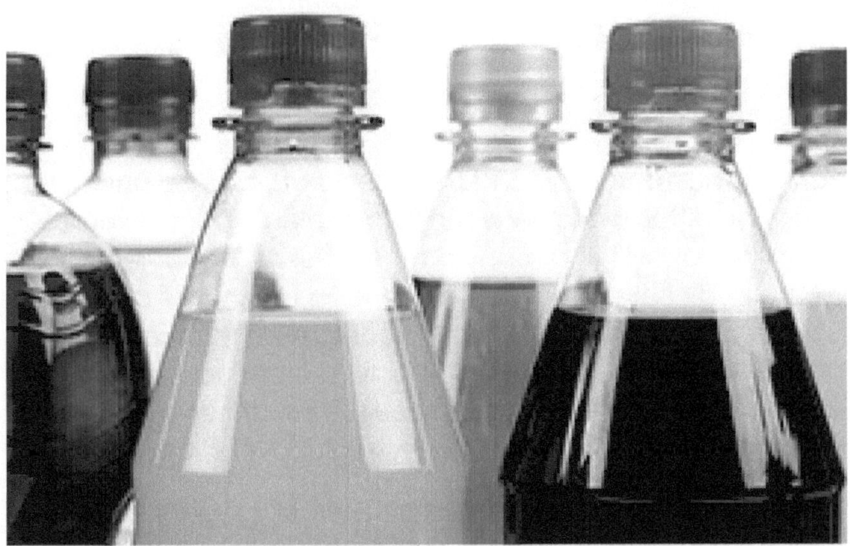

An in depth study on sugar reveals that it is a quite refined form of carbohydrate, same as potatoes, white rice or flour. However, it creates higher impact on obesity and diabetes than these foods. This is because the perils of sugar are enormous and one of the reasons for it being hazardous is that it is a refined form of carbohydrate. Secondly, the principal element that makes sugar toxic is the fructose. The composition of sucrose involves equal portions of fructose and glucose. The glucose part is responsible for elevating blood sugars and driving the response of insulin, whereas fructose has no such role. Fructose does not promote a rise in blood sugars. Hence, it is known for the low figure in glycemic index. Additionally, fructose creates a little increase in insulin levels than glucose. People for several years, have considered fructose as a mild sweetener. This idea is further supported when the sweetening agent in fruits was found to be fructose. Apparently, this natural sugar in fruit, which does not increase glucose levels in blood, looks quite healthy. But in reality, when you study the subject thoroughly, the harmful effects of fructose will leave you astonished.

HOW FRUCTOSE AFFECTS YOU ADVERSELY?

You can never understand the effects of fructose unless you know the differences between fructose and glucose, and surprisingly, you will find many differences. As explained earlier, all the body cells can utilize glucose. In fact, there are cells in your body that can only use glucose. An example in this regard is the red blood cells. Similarly, skeletal muscles are another important example that requires instant energy for body movement and so they prefer using glucose.

Now, fructose cannot be used by any cell in your body to get energy. Different studies have shown that fructose is not absorbed in the gut of human body. However, if glucose is present, then it can improve the poor absorption of fructose and the quantity of fructose absorbed increases. As far as absorption of glucose is concerned, unlike fructose, it needs insulin to get absorbed at maximum level. Once absorbed, glucose can move freely throughout your body to be used as energy, whereas fructose, which is avoided by most of the cells, keeps piling up in the liver where it is metabolized.

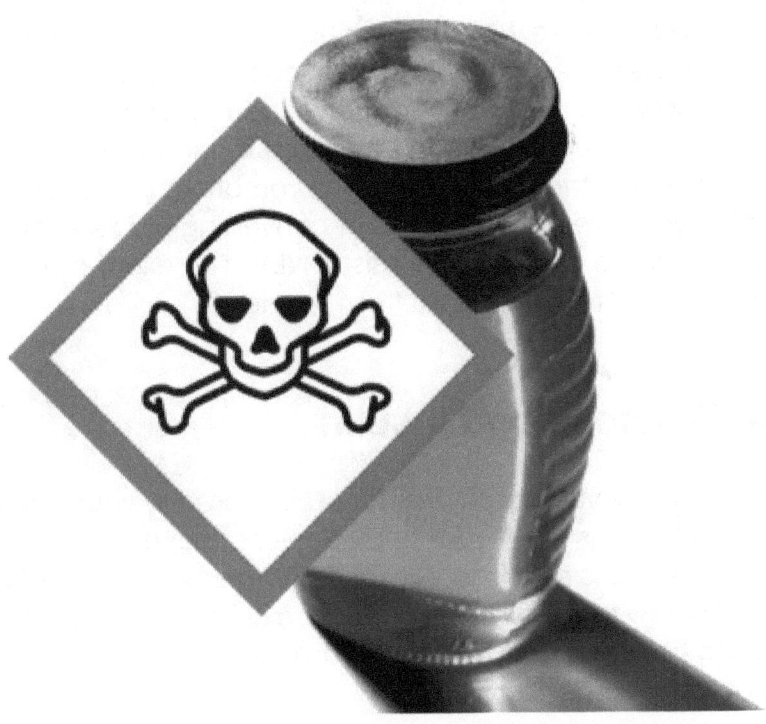

Fructose is converted into fructose-1-phosphate quickly without any limitations. When you intake extensive amount of glucose, your body acts naturally to limit its amount, hence preventing unnecessary overloading of your body's metabolic system. This whole process is not applicable in case of fructose. As your intake of food rises, your metabolism also increases. The food coverts into glucose, glycogen and lactate; all of them get concentrated in your liver. The ingestion of fructose leads to the formation of acetyl-CoA that is required for the synthesis of fatty acids. This statement implies that high fructose level turns into fat in your liver, consequently making it a fatty liver.

Fatty liver is extremely important in developing insulin resistance in your liver. What actually happens is, insulin is produced when you consume any food. This insulin enables the glucose in your body to get stored as energy packets that can be used in future when you do not eat anything. Some of the glucose is stored in the form of glycogen for a limited time period. However, liver can store glycogen in small amount. The remaining glucose has to be stored in the form of fat. Thus, you can say that insulin helps in promoting the generation of fat in your liver. This process of converting glucose into fat is called as de novo lipogenesis (DNL). The exact meaning of the term is "to produce fat from the new".

● Fructose and Insulin

The energy you obtain from food is stored in your body with the help of insulin. If your body does not have enough insulin, the process is reversed. Glycogen converts itself into glucose, and a new form of fat is produced to energize your body. If the gaps between fasting and feed periods are balanced, then net fat becomes zero.

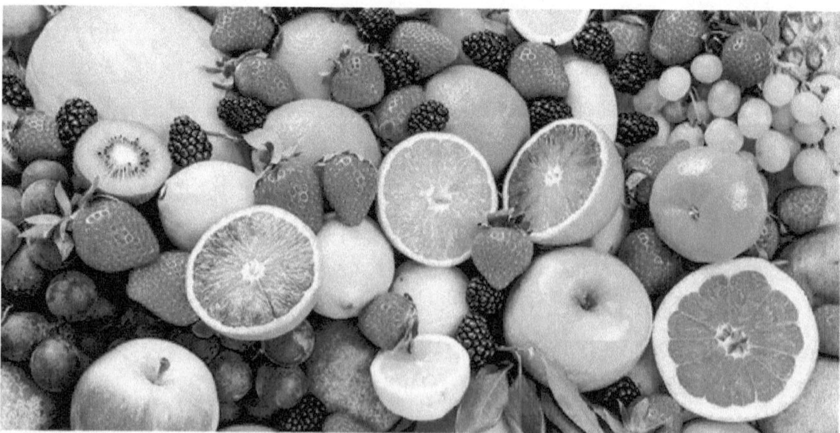

Insulin tries to inject more fat into the liver that is already fatty. The role of insulin here is similar to inflating balloon that is already overinflated. This means it becomes difficult for insulin to push energy derived from food into the liver. Since, the usual amount of insulin fails to force the sugar into your liver, the need of insulin increases to push the same quantity of sugar into your fatty liver. This process is known as "insulin resistance". Your body becomes resistant to whatever efforts are made by insulin.

Another issue with the overly fatty liver is that higher insulin levels are needed for keeping fat and sugar together. When insulin levels decrease, sugar is released in the blood, thus resulting high sugar levels in your bloodstream.

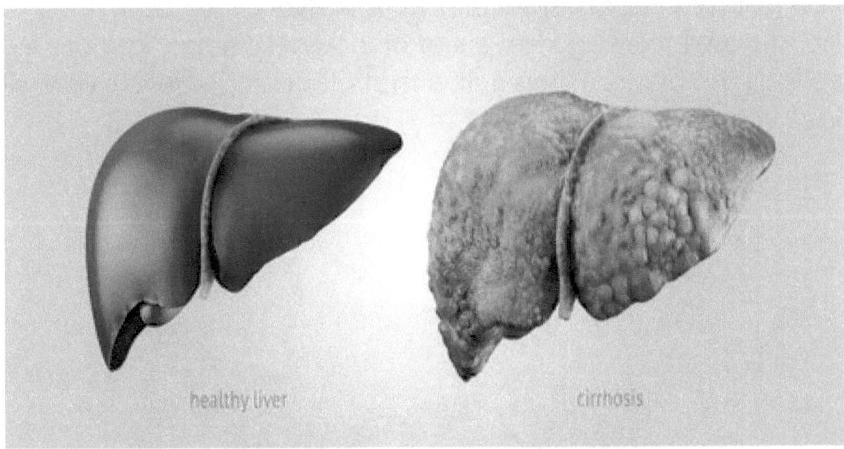

This is disliked by your body and it opposes this phenomenon with elevated levels of insulin. Hence, you can conclude that insulin resistance causes insulin levels to rise further, that in turn, promote the storage of fat and sugar into your liver. Consequently, more fat is over-crammed in the fatty liver, leading to more insulin resistance. The cycle continues and the ultimate result is obesity of the body, or "hyperinsulinemia".

● What is Hyperinsulinemia?

When there is an abnormal increase in the levels of insulin in your bloodstream, this condition is called **"Hyperinsulin-emia"**. This disease is linked with type 2 diabetes; however technically, you cannot regard it as a type of diabetes. This condition is one of the factors leading to obesity, metabolic syndrome and insulin resistance.

If your body develops insulin **resistance,** glucose accumulates in the blood. As glucose becomes inaccessible for your body to get fueled, the cells turn into starvation mode, and you get thirsty or hungry all the time. Now your body tries to bring down the sugar levels in blood by eliminating more insulin in the blood. The result is that blood sugar levels as well insulin rises a lot.

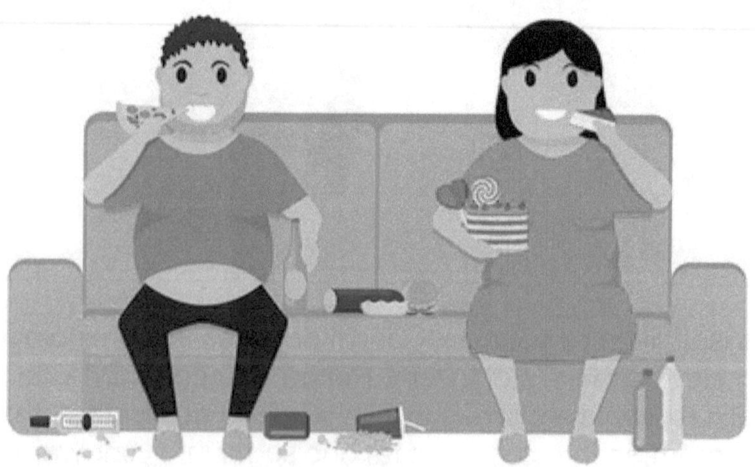

Excessive insulin lowers blood sugar, which is being circulated in the whole body, and so hypoglycemia becomes a prominent indicator of its existence. This condition specially appears in infants who are given birth by mothers with a history of uncontrollable diabetes. Few other signs of hyperinsulinemia are; high sugar levels due to insulin resistance, elevated triglyceride and blood cholesterol levels, increased blood pressure, weight gain, fatigue, problems in shedding weight, and a lot of cravings for sugar/ carbohydrate.

OBESITY AND HIGH INSULIN LEVELS

As discussed earlier, when high amount of fructose is metabolized, fatty liver is formed, and this fatty liver is the leading cause in developing insulin resistance. High insulin levels result in obesity. Any imbalance between protective factors; like vinegar and fiber, and dietary factors, such as fattening or carbohydrates, contributes obesity. Then, another aspect that needs to be considered is, insulin resistance creates a time-dependent effect that alters insulin levels. All this forms a vicious cycle where increased insulin levels enhance insulin resistance and then again insulin level rises further. As the cycle becomes long, it gets worsened.

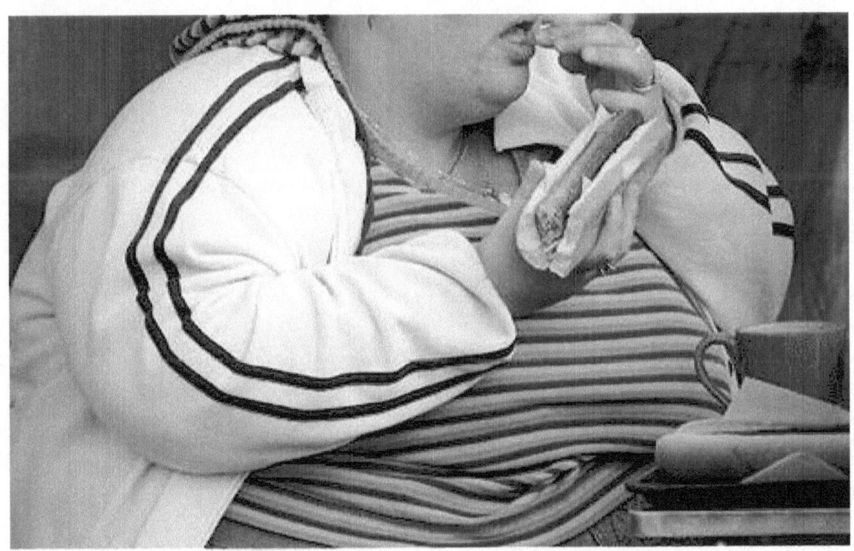

Fructose is another element that develops insulin resistance apart from high levels of insulin. This has been explained in detail while describing fatty liver induction and hepatic insulin resistance. This makes it clear that why sugar appears fattening. Sugar triggers insulin and of course, insulin resistance. Overtime the continuous consumption of sugar results in higher levels of insulin, which lead to obesity. Therefore, it can be said that sugars are not simply refined carbohydrates, in fact more harmful than that.

Therefore, the conclusion we draw is that you can avoid getting over-weight by cutting our sugar from your diet. In addition, never replace sugar with sweeteners as they are also bad for your health.

04

CURE OBESITY AND TYPE 2 DIABETES NATURALLY

If you check the internet, you will see many sources, making fake promises of providing magical foods and drugs that will make you fit and smart miraculously. Herbalist offering herbs such as Capsiberry, Sea Buckthorn, saffron extract, African mango, Garcinia Cambogia, Yacon syrup, green coffee extract and Raspberry ketones are some of them. But do they really work? Are miracle cures a reality? The truth is heart breaking and the whole phenomena of a miracle weight loss is completely bogus and absurd.

● Avoid Miracle Cures

We already know this deep in our hearts that it does not work. We have been eating herbs and plants since 1000 of years, so how it is possible that all of a sudden in 2015, a plant or herb can melt away your all body fat? Thus, it is merely stupidity. In fact, the idea of having superfoods also does not work. Having superfoods mean that you have meals that can automatically make you extraordinarily healthy in just a matter of days, which is ridiculous. Our mind has been manipulated to believe that a plant from a certain forest or a seed from specific place is enough to beat diabetes and obesity. In the mid of the 19th century, people do not use to rely on eating seeds to cure obesity, neither do they take processed foods, instead they used to eat unprocessed foods, such as fish, olive oil, vegetables, fruits and nuts. Thus, diabetes and obesity was not a major issue then. The thing is we need to understand the cause of weight gain to avoid obesity. Secondly, we should stop relying on miracles to cure diabetes or obesity.

WHAT NOT TO EAT

As we all clearly know that insulin is the major player in the development of obesity, now our focus should be to cure it first. Since insulin causes us to gain weight, thus our aim is to first decrease insulin. Also. Keep in mind, when you are obese, it is not because of imbalance of calories in your body, but it is due to hormonal changes. Therefore, getting rid of obesity is not simple as increasing the consumption of vegetables, fruits and fibers or lowering processed foods, sugars and carbs from your diet, in fact, you need to work on lowering insulin. So what increases insulin? There are few factors that contribute in it, one of them includes, the meals we take. There are specific foods that result increase insulin in your body, whereas, there also some foods that decrease its levels. So, this takes us to the conclusion that we should know what to add and what to limit in our daily diet to stop insulin spikes.

● Reduce the Intake of Added Sugars

It is quite clear that the first step in any weight loss program is to decrease the intake of added sugar. In the long term, sugar is specifically dangerous, as it spikes your insulin levels very quickly. Sugar contains both fructose and glucose equally.

Glucose is actually a six ringed sugar, which is present in your blood. Almost every cell in the body can utilize glucose. For instance, it acts as a major source of energy in the brain. Likewise, muscle cells derive it from the bloodstream for an instant boost of energy. Liver stores glucose in different forms like glycogen. When your body is under stress, glucose is released for boosting energy quickly. In fact, glucose keeps circulating throughout your body without any limitations.

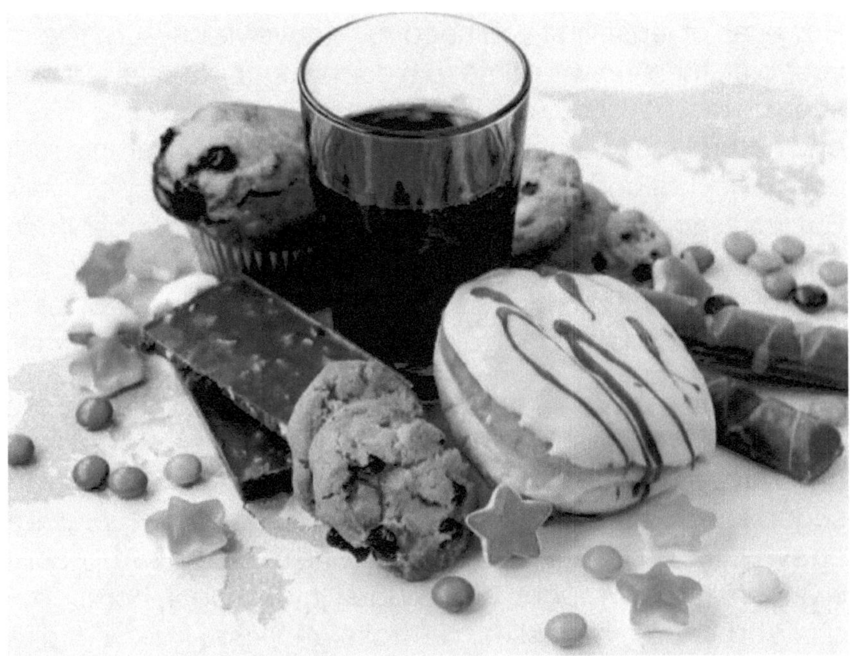

On the contrary, fructose is a five ringed sugar, which is a natural ingredient in fruits. The Liver metabolizes this sugar and it no more circulates as fructose as your body is incapable of using fructose in its original form. For instance, your muscles and brain have no ability to use fructose. That is the reason why, the ingestion of fructose does not considerably alter the sugar levels in blood.

Glucose stimulates insulin directly and increase sugar levels in your blood, whereas. Fructose has a direct contribution in the liver causing insulin resistance. This is an understood phenomena that insulin resistance results in greater insulin levels.

Thus, one of the most important foods that you immediately need to restrict from your diet is sugar. They have no nutritional value for your body. However, the issue is that it is not easy to avoid sugars because sugar is in almost every processed food and sometimes we take foods without even realizing it has sugar in it.

However, at least, first you need to remove visible sugar from your diet, then we will come to hidden sugar. No need to add sugar in any beverage or food. There are several unprocessed and natural foods as well that contain sugar, for example milk and fruits that comprise of lactose and fructose respectively. But, you should be qualifies enough to differentiate between natural and added sugar. Even though fruits have sugar, but they also provide nutritional value, such as vitamins and fibers and all this act as a shield to overcome the impact of fructose.

There are several other names as well for sugar and these are labelled with different names, so a consumer gets confused and buys it, without knowing that he is actually consuming sugar. These names include agave nectar, palm syrup, golden syrup, malt syrup, maple syrup, cane and corn syrup, corn sweetener, brown sugar, cane sugar, invert sugar, honey, hydrolyzed starch, molasses, dextrose, maltose, fructose, glucose and sucrose. These are some of the tricks to hide the sugar.

Similarly, dipping sauces, such as sweet and sour sauce, hoisin sauce, honey garlic sauce, plum sauce and barbeque has an immense amount of sugar. You should also avoid commercial condiments and salad dressings, such as ketchup. The rule is simple, if the product is in in packaging, it has sugar in it.

DESSERTS

You can easily identify and eliminate most of the desserts from your diet. Such foods contain high sugar content in different forms in which artificial flavors are added to give a unique taste, for instance; puddings, cakes, pies, cookies, ice-cream, mousses, candy, sorbets and candy bars. Now, you must be thinking that what options are now left if you are craving for desserts. The best way is to consume desserts that are preferred in traditional societies like seasonal fruits that are taken from locally grown farms. You can take a bowl of strawberries or cherries with creamy sauce or lemon juice as topping to satisfy your sweet tooth. Likewise, if you take a hand full of nuts and mix with cheese without adding any sugar, it is also a great combination of food and can be treated as a dessert. Then, taking dark chocolate that has at least 70% of cacao is a also a good treat. This is because, cocoa beans in chocolate are not sweet naturally and do not have sugar, unlike milk chocolates that contain high amount of sugar. White or milk chocolate contains more sugar compared to dark chocolate or chocolates that have mild sweetness. Dark chocolate also has a high amount of fiber as well as antioxidants like flavanols and polyphenols.

It is an accepted fact that no celebration is complete without food, whether it is a wedding, birthday, Christmas, graduation etc. Since celebrations come occasionally, and so they are special where food is enjoyed by everyone. Dessert is an important element in any celebration, and obviously they are not eaten every day. However, if your primary goal is to lose weight, you need to avoid sugar completely. If you are thinking to replace sugar with some artificial sweeteners then it is a bad idea, as insulin increases due to sweeteners as well, just like sugar. Both of these result in obesity.

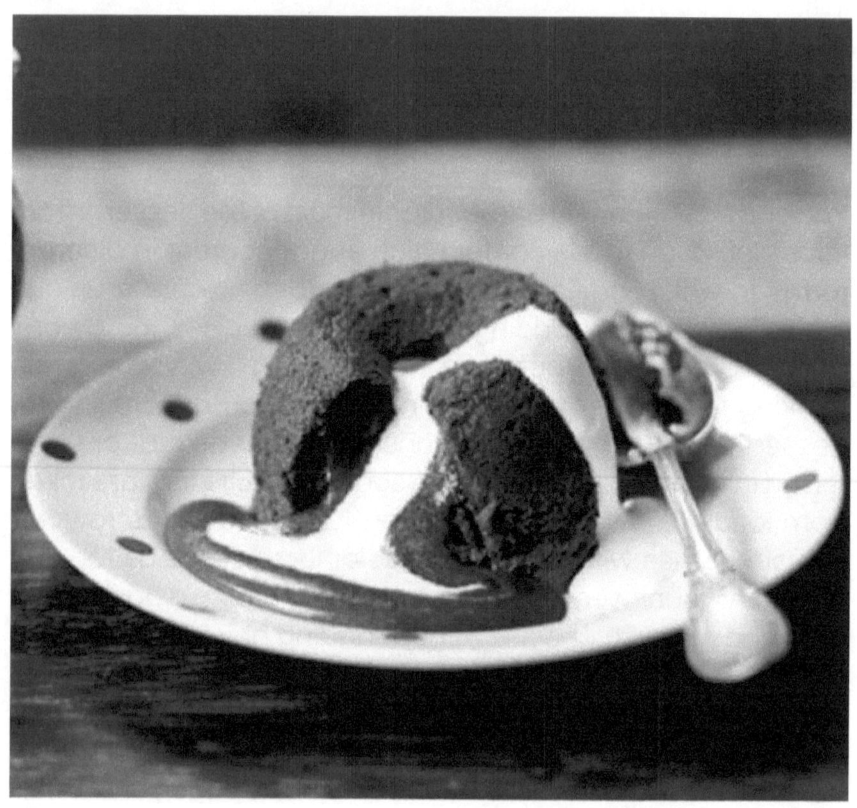

MYTH ABOUT BREAKFAST

Undoubtedly, breakfast is one such meal of the day that has been in discussion for several years by health practitioners and advisors. You must have heard since childhood that you need to eat something when you leave bed every morning as your body needs energy at the start of the day. If someone skips breakfast, people make him feel guilty as if he/she has committed a major health crime. You must realize that break-fast is just a meal and not "a very important meal" that cannot be skipped.

It is not a big issue if you skip breakfast, but the main issue is eating foods in breakfast that are mostly desserts in disguise and comprise of the high amount of sugar and processed car-bohydrates. This is especially true for breakfast cereals pre-pared for kids. According to a study, they contain 45% more sugar compared to cereals prepared for adults.

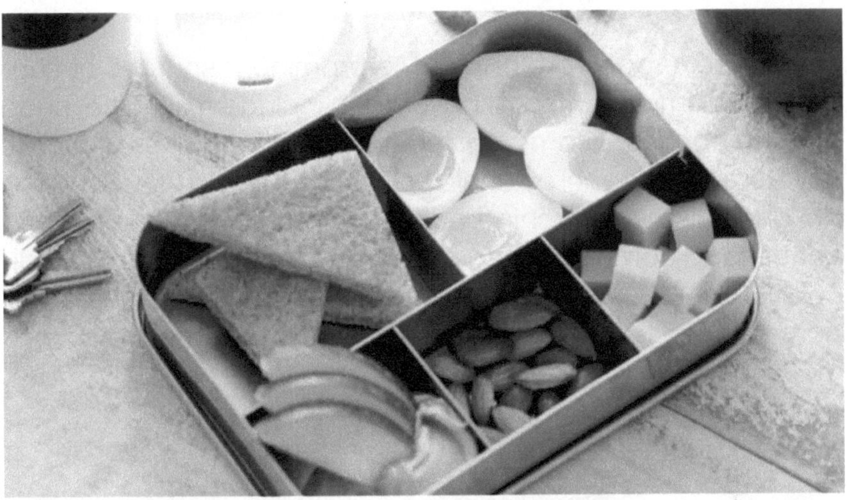

Breakfast cereals for children come after cookies, ice-creams, candies and sugar drinks in the list of foods that offer dietary sugar. Although, the other mentioned items are des-serts, breakfast cereals are considered as healthy meal and are promoted extensively through marketing. Nevertheless, whole grains addition in your diet improves your health, but it also enhances sugar level in your body.

Now, the question that pops up in mind is that what can you eat at breakfast? If you do not feel hungry, you need not eat anything. No harm will be done to your body if you directly take a meal at noon with a piece of grilled fish and fresh salad. Sim-ilarly, if you are hungry in the morning, you can eat something healthy and again, it is just a meal, like other meals of the day. It is often observed that when you are in a rush early morning, you go for convenient foods like heavily processed or sugary foods. This leads to unhealthy eating habits. You must eat un-processed, whole foods every time no matter whether you are in a rush or not. If you are short of time, then do not eat instead of consuming sugary, processed foods.

BEVERAGES

Sugary beverages are one of the prominent sources of sug-ar. The examples of such beverages include fruit juice, soda pop, smoothies, vitamin water, fruit punch, shakes, flavored milk, lemonade, energy drink, cold-coffee and so on. Similarly, hot drinks like moccachino, hot chocolate, sweetened tea and coffee, also come under sugar beverages category. Then, al-coholic drinks also have a major amount of sugar, for instance, hard lemonade, coolers, flavored wines, cider beers etc.

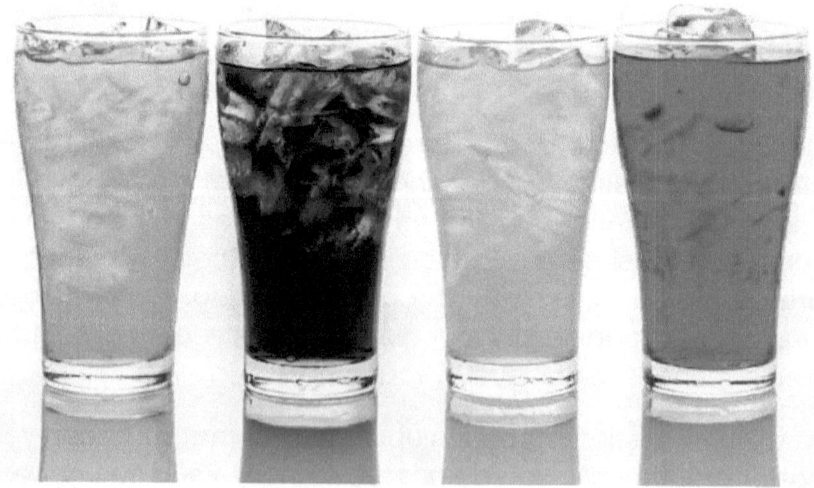

Traditional obeverages that are widely consumed all over the world have high sugar content as well, like margaritas, pi-na-coladas, daiquiris, dessert wines, sweet sherries, liqueurs and ice wines. All these examples leave a question mark as to what can you drink? It is best to drink plain water. You can add slices of orange, lemon or cucumber to make yourself more refreshed.

WHEAT

Wheat is consumed throughout the world as one of the major domesticated foods for centuries. Your body converts wheat into glucose easily compared to other food items. Wheat is also a significant source of gluten and this gluten generates exorphins in your body. When gluten is digested, certain substances that are similar to morphine are produced, which may get absorbed in the blood and brain and so are considered addictive.

According to several surveys, people are of the view that they become addicted to pasta and bread. Certain other bakery items and snacks are also flour based like cookies, macaroni cheese and cakes. There are people who are addicted to eating such items without caring that how much these can affect their health and body weight.

Today, wheat is the most powerful food item that enhances body weight. When you increase wheat intake your Body Mass Index also rises. Wheat intake is also associated with coronary diseases. Wheat consumption in excessive amount is a great issue because:

- It offers low nutritional value

- Its processing eliminates the high amount of vitamins and fiber

- Recent milling techniques accelerate the digestion process, thus enhancing glycemic effect

- It is has high amount of amylopectin.

- It may make you addicted to it

It is not necessary that all carbohydrates result in obesity. But, refined grains like flour definitely promote obesity. Hence, if you are trying to lose weight, you must decrease intake of refined grains, especially wheat.

● Cure Diabetes Naturally

Diabetes type 2 is one of the popular diseases that is very common nowadays. It is a chronic disease that slowly damages your body organs. Even though, medicines play an important role in helping to control sugar, but continuous consumption of medicines has some harmful side effects for your health. Some of the popular drugs for sugar include Rosiglitazone, Glyburide and Metformin. The first few months of taking drugs show great improvement, but after sometime, sugar again starts to increase and then you have to switch to different drugs. People with diabetes usually start with Metformin, then doctors prescribe to take both Glyburide and Metformin, when one drug is not helpful and finally you have to take 3 to 4 drugs for this issue. When all these drugs stop working, your doctor asks you to take insulin artificially, and increases its dosage with time.

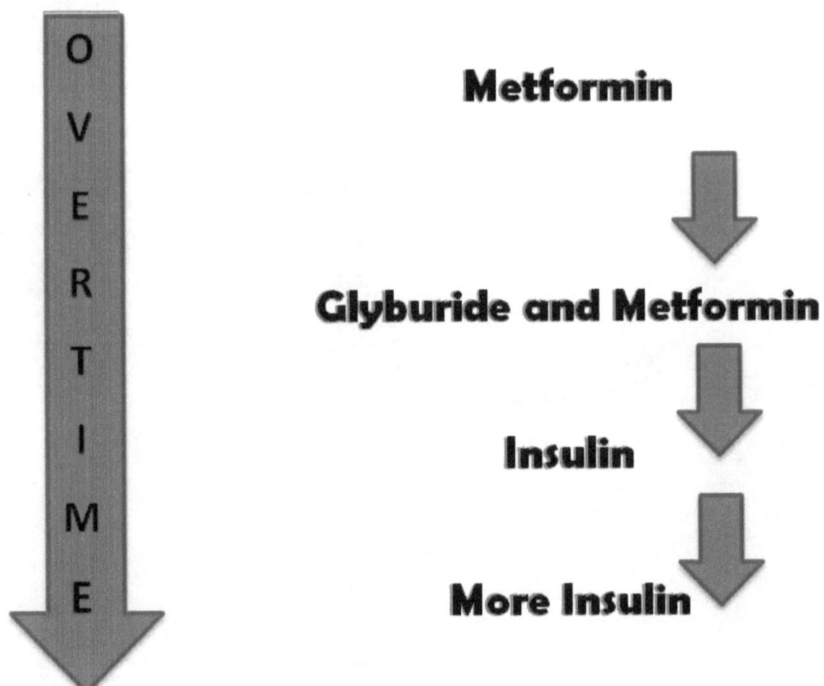

The above chart also shows that if the patient is taking Metformin in small amounts, this means he has mild diabetes and if he is taking a large amount of insulin, this indicates, his diabetes has gone worse. Over time, your diabetes gets worse only, no matter what people tell you. Your sugar level fluctuates, but your diabetes is just getting worse. People usually get confused and think diabetes and sugar are the same thing, but actually, it is not. These are entirely different things. Insulin resistance is the cause of diabetes and sugars are just a sign that you have insulin resistance.

For example, simply, think of an infection. You have an infection in your kidney and the symptom this infection shows is fever, so what will be your priority? Is it to treat fever or infection? Of course, your doctor will work to cure infection. You would require antibiotic to treat infection. Same is the story of diabetes. Your disease is all about insulin resistance and here the symptom is presence of sugar in your blood. The drugs are working just to control sugar and working only on symptoms, instead of the cause. In this way, this disease is only getting worse.

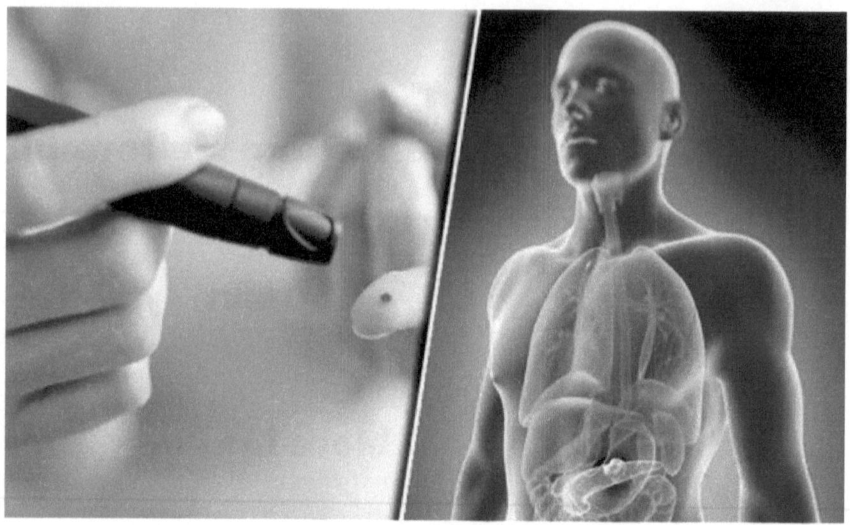

In the end, even if you get successful to control your sugar, it will make no difference on your disease. You still have to face the complications of diabetes, such as kidney disease, eye disease, heart disease and strokes. Because all this time your focus has been to treat the symptom, instead of the disease.

Here the key player is insulin. This is because when the levels of insulin becomes high, it results in insulin resistance and then ultimately in type 2 diabetes. Therefore, it is essential to decrease insulin resistance in order to improve diabetes and promote weight loss

One of the major reasons that people with type 2 diabetes are obese is because their body produces higher levels of insulin and insulin plays an important role in storing body fat. Therefore, insulin is responsible for both insulin resistance and weight gain.

Insulin tries to inject more fat into the liver that is already fatty. The role of insulin here is similar to inflating balloon that is already overinflated. This means it becomes difficult for insulin to push energy derived from food into the liver. Since, the usual amount of insulin fails to force the sugar into your liver, the need of insulin increases to push the same quantity of sugar into your fatty liver. This process is known as "insulin resistance". Your body becomes resistant to whatever efforts are made by insulin.

Hence, you can conclude that insulin resistance causes insulin levels to rise further, that in turn, promote the storage of fat and sugar into your liver. Consequently, more fat is over-crammed in the fatty liver, leading to more insulin resistance.

When you take more insulin, your body develops resistance to it and because of this your body get a higher level of insulin. The greater level of insulin, the more your body becomes resistant to it. This cycle goes on. Thus, insulin treatment becomes ineffective. In fact, it is making your diabetes worse. With the intake of insulin, your diabetes gets worse. The problem is people do not understand this and keep on taking insulin.

Diabetes is a dietary disease, it can't be cured with antibiotics or insulin, but from diets and intermittent fasting.

What intermittent fasting does is, it helps you in cutting down the number of calories by reducing meals that you take per day. It is an acceptable fact that quitting eating for some time is highly convenient compared to eating less.

When you restrict your meal frequency, this reduces insulin to lower levels in your body, and give it some time get activated to the ketosis mode. The term "ketosis" can be defined as a state where fat is used to derive energy instead of sugar, thus promoting weight-loss.

People have been fasting since years. It is one of the major pillars in almost every religion. The practice of fasting is very healthy because it keeps your insulin levels down. Another way to cure diabetes is to have refined carbs in your diet. This is because carbohydrates increase your insulin levels. Thus, if you want to treat diabetes naturally, combine low-carb diet with intermittent fasting for amazing results.

05: TYPES OF FATS

We usually hear that some types of fats are good for you and some are bad for you. But what are actually bad and good types of fats? This chapter uncovers this question.

Monounsaturated and polyunsaturated fats are good for you, trans fats are bad for you, while saturated fats somewhere lie between the good and bad fats.

People when hear the word 'Fat' get scared and want to erase it completely from their diet, as they think that fat is the major culprit in increasing their weight. If you also think that switching to low-fat foods is the solution, then you are at mistake, as this shift will not make you healthy, as you might be cutting back on fats that are healthy for you.

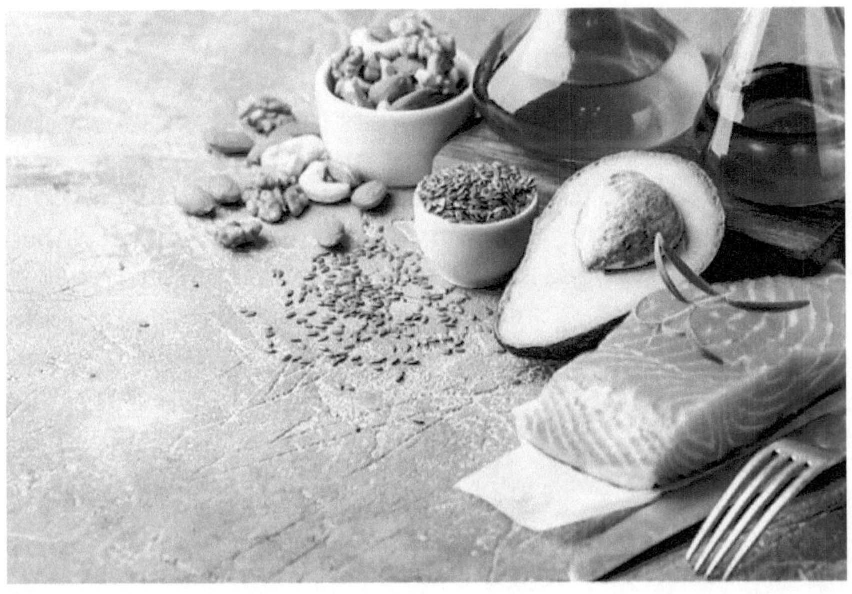

Your body requires fat as it is the main source of energy. Fats help in absorbing some minerals and vitamins in your body. It is required for building cell membranes. Besides, it is essential for inflammation, muscle movement, and blood clotting. Poly-unsaturated and monounsaturated fats are good fats. The bad ones are trans made (industrial made fats).

Even though, all fats have the same chemical structure, which is a chain of carbon atoms attached to hydrogen atoms. But, the shape and length of carbon and quantity of hydrogen atoms attached with the carbon atoms make it different from another. These little differences in structure result in major differences in function and form.

BAD TYPE OF FATS (TRANS FATS)

Trans fats are considered as the worst type of dietary fat. This fat is basically a byproduct of hydrogenation (a process which is utilized for converting healthy oils into solids as well as to protect them from reeking). There is no safe limit of consuming trans fat, neither it provides any benefit for your body. In fact, in the US, trans fats are banned officially.

In the start of the 20th century, trans fats were majorly found in vegetable shortening and solid margarines. However, with time, when food makers learned new methods to use vegetable oils (partially hydrogenated), they started appearing in all sorts of categories in foods, from fast-food French fries to commercial pastries and cookies. But, currently, many countries have banned trans fats.

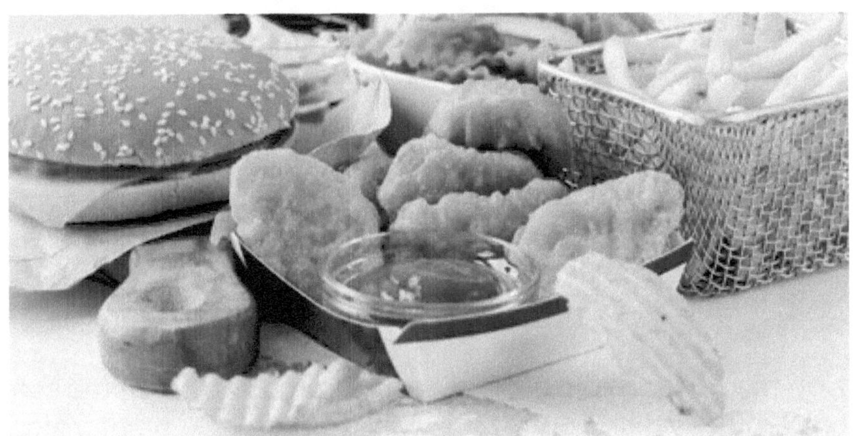

The major side effect of having trans fat in your diet is that it decreases the good cholesterol (HDL) from your bloodstream and instead increases harmful cholesterol (LDL).

This ultimately creates inflammation, which may lead to several chronic conditions, such as diabetes, stroke and heart diseases. Insulin resistance is also caused by trans fat, which increases the probability of having type 2 diabetes. Even consuming a little amount of trans fats can harm your health. Studies show that the chances of heart disease increase by 23 percent for every 2% of calories consumed daily from trans fat.

● Saturated Fats (In-Between)

If we talk about saturated fats, these are solid at room temperature, such as cooled bacon grease. The major sources of saturated fat are:

- Coconut Oil

- Cheese

- Whole-Milk Dairy Foods

- Whole Milk

- Red Meat

- Baked Foods That Are Prepared Commercially

Here, when we say saturated, it means the quantity of hydrogen atoms around each carbon atom. Each carbon atom is saturated with hydrogen. It holds as many hydrogens as possible.

Now the question arises whether it is harmful to consume saturated fat? When you have meals that are rich in saturated fats, this increases your total cholesterol, which include your both good and bad cholesterol. This, in result prompts blockages to develop in the heart's arteries. Thus, health practitioners recommend to have a limited amount saturated fat (up to 10 percent of total calories in a day).

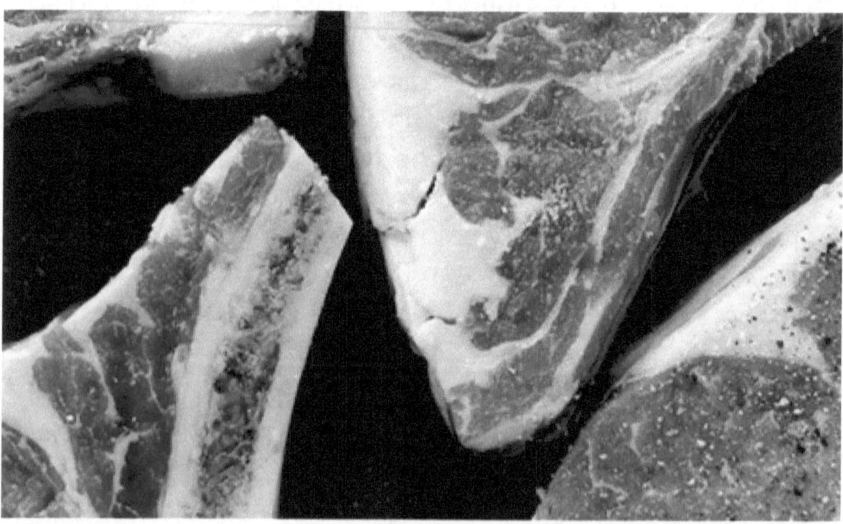

There are many recent studies that have proved the connection between heart disease and saturated fats and if we replace saturated fat meals with polyunsaturated foods (carbohydrates containing high fiber or vegetable oils), then the probability of having heart disease decreases.

● Good Polyunsaturated And Monounsaturated Fats

Mainly, we get good fats from fish, seeds, nut and vegetables. These fat are different from saturated and trans fats because their carbon chains have fewer hydrogens attached with them. Good fats, when they are at room temperature, they are in the liquid form. These fat are divided into two main categories, named as polyunsaturated and monounsaturated fats.

POLYUNSATURATED FATS: The liquid oil that you use for cooking is a polyunsaturated fat. Some of the common examples include safflower oil, sunflower oil and corn oil. These fat are also known as essential fats. This means your body is not capable of making this fat and these are required for general body functions. Therefore, it is a must to get these fat from meals.

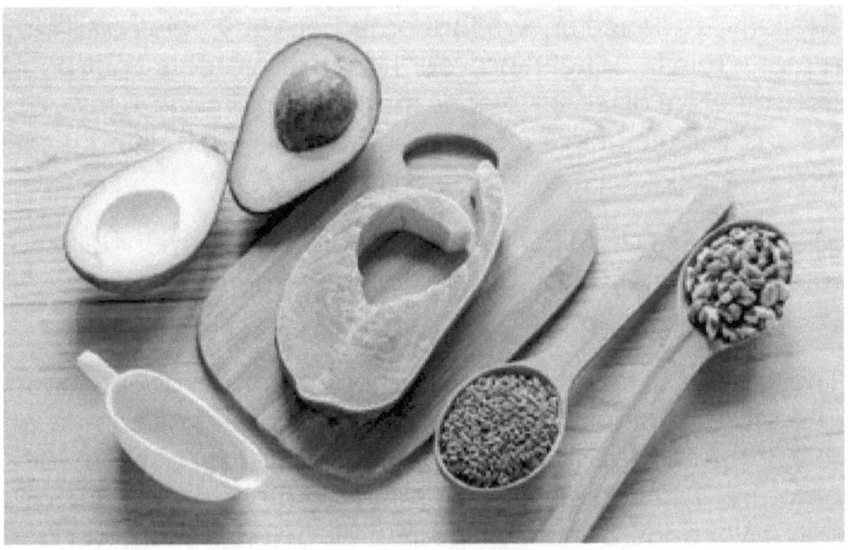

The responsibility of polyunsaturated fats is to build the covering of nerves and cell membranes. Besides, they are also required for inflammation, muscle movement and blood clotting. There are two or more than two double bonds present in the carbon chain of a polyunsaturated fat. It has two types, which include omega-6 fatty acids and omega-3 fatty acids. Both the fatty acids offer amazing health benefits.

When we eat polyunsaturated fats instead of highly refined carbohydrates or saturated fats, it improves the overall cholesterol profile by reducing harmful LDL cholesterol. It is also helpful in lowering triglycerides. Some of the major sources of omega-3 fatty acids are unhydrogenated soybean oil, canola oil, walnuts, flaxseeds and fatty fish, which include sardines, mackerel and salmon.

With the intake of omega-3 fatty acids, you can prevent as well as cure heart stroke and disease. Polyunsaturated fats lower triglycerides, raise HDL, reduce blood pressure and protect lethal heart rhythms from occurring. Those people who are suffering from rheumatoid arthritis, polyunsaturated fats decrease their need to take steroids.

Similarly, evidence shows that omega-6 fatty acids also play a major role in benefitting your health. It protects your heart from different diseases. Foods that contain omega-6 fatty acids and linoleic acid include vegetable oils such as corn oils, walnut, sunflower, soybean and safflower.

MONOUNSATURATED FATS: You are having monounsaturated fat when you are at an Italian restaurant and you dip your bread in olive oil.

These types of fat have a one carbon-to-carbon double bond. Therefore, it has less number of hydrogen atoms as compared to a saturated fat. These are also in liquid state at room temperature. The rich sources of monounsaturated fats include nuts, avocados, canola oil, peanut oil, olive oil, sunflower and safflower oils.

There is no limit to take monounsaturated fats, in fact, it is recommended to take as much polyunsaturated fats and monounsaturated fats to replace trans and saturated fats.

WHY FAT DOES NOT MAKE YOU FAT?

Most of the people have this misconception that if they are consuming fats, it will make them fat. This part of the ebook will clear this misconception.

When we consume lots of carbohydrates, it is converted into sugar, which later on spikes insulin (the fat storing hormone). It does not matter that you are overweight or not, insulin drives all energy available in your bloodstream into your fat cells, specifically, around your belly, also known as organ fat or visceral fat. All this incites your brain to eat more.

Moreover, when we try to exercise and restrict calories (a common method used by people to lose weight), all of a sudden, your body becomes alarmed and fear that you are starving. Because of this, you feel tired and your body tries to conserve energy. This makes you to eat more, as you become hungry.

Experiments and studies show that those who eat diets with high fats, have a faster metabolism, while people who eat high carb and low fat diets have a slow metabolism, more belly fat because of a spike in insulin.

However, you have to be careful while consuming fats that they should be healthy fats (either polyunsaturated or monounsaturated fats). The intake of good fats helps in improving your metabolism and taste preferences.

06

AN OVERVIEW OF INTERMITTENT FASTING

WHAT DO YOU MEAN BY INTERMITTENT FASTING?

When you fast for intermittent period, then it is called "Intermittent Fasting" (IF). This implies a pattern of taking food in which the cycle revolves around the phase of food intake and the phase of voluntary fasting during a single day, or week or some other defined time period.

If you put it in simple words, you can say that intermittent fasting is to control when to take food and when not. The time period when you stop taking any food or drink (apart from water), is known as "fasting window", and the remaining period is known as "eating window".

Now, it purely depends on you about what should be the duration of your eating window or fasting that is the schedule of your intermittent fasting.

HOW INTERMITTENT FASTING WORKS FOR YOUR BODY?

Intermittent Fasting comprises of two elements: first is limiting calories, which means consuming less calories than required by your body. Second is a reduction in frequency of meals that is the number of snacks or meal you take per day.

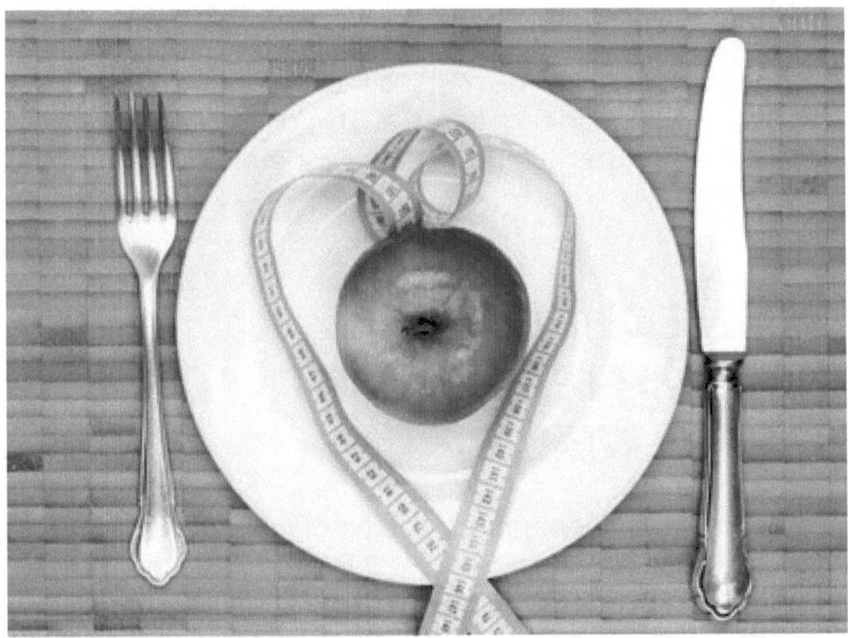

Usually, an adult follows a dietary routine as taking a breakfast early morning like 8am, then lunch after 12pm that is at noon, snack around 4pm, then dinner at 8 pm. Later, his mind does not allow him to go to bed without eating anything and so he prefers taking some snack at 11pm. This makes a total of 5 meals over a period of fifteen hours. When you do not control the portions of your meals strictly, you end up consuming more calories than needed by your body on that particular day, and this contributes to weight gain.

Above all, your body keeps working throughout the day to digest the food and is left with no time to perform activities for recovery. When you set a schedule for intermittent fasting, you minimize the frequency of meals that should be taken throughout the day. This makes it difficult for you to take three big meals and two snacks.

When following any intermittent fasting schedule you are reducing the meal frequency throughout your day, making it simply harder to eat 3 big meals and 2 snacks in a time period, which is less either twice or thrice the earlier time span. This change in diet pattern decreases the chances to exceed the calorie consumption requirement. This also offers more time to your body for performing recovery operations like autophagy.

THE MECHANISM OF INTERMITTENT FASTING FOR LOSING WEIGHT

In order to get a deep understanding of the mechanism of intermittent fasting, you must first go through the basics of diet and nutrition. This can be explained in simple words as, the food you consume breaks down into molecules and gets absorbed into your blood, hence feeding your body cells. Few of these molecules appear as net carbohydrates, which mean subtracting fiber from total carbohydrates in the meal. The net carbohydrates are then converted into sugar or glucose and these are used as energy to fuel our body.

Insulin is needed by your body for using sugar to get energy. Pancreas in your body is responsible for producing insulin every time you intake carbohydrates. Sugar that is in excessive amount and is not consumed, is stored as fat. This fat is used later to get energy when no sugar is left.

If you do not want to accumulate heavy amount of fat in your body and gain lot of weight, then you must spend all the energy you obtain by taking food. It has been observed that mostly lavish lifestyles of people minimize their chances to increase movement throughout the day. The biggest example in this regard is the office workers who spend at least 80% of their day sitting on chair.

Now the question arises that what can be done to avoid weight-gain or lose excess weight? One of the ways is to make efforts to increase energy consumption of your body by increasing physical activities, which include regular workout and taking part in sports. Then, another method is reducing food intake than the requirement of your body to get energy on a certain day. This creates a calorie deficit and helps in achieving your target.

HERE COMES THE ROLE OF INTERMITTENT FASTING!

What intermittent fasting does is, it helps you in cutting down the number of calories by reducing meals that you take per day. It is an acceptable fact that quitting eating for some time is highly convenient compared to eating less.

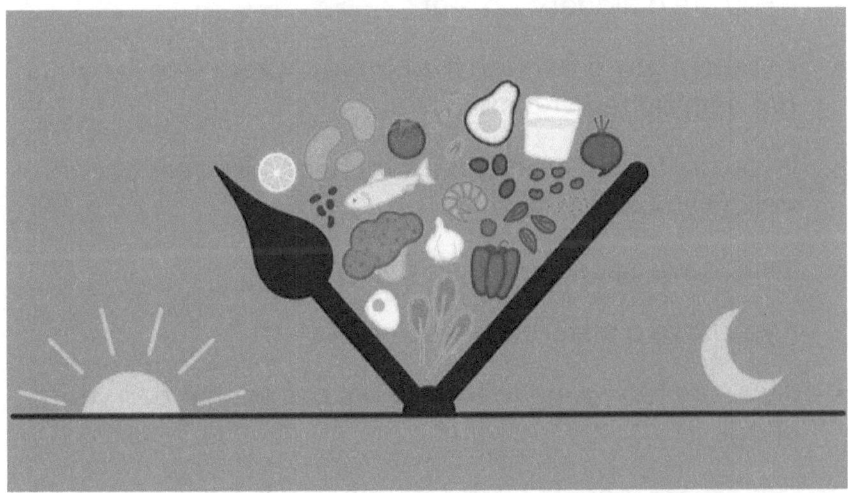

When you restrict your meal frequency, this reduces insulin to lower levels in your body, and give it some time get activated to the ketosis mode. The term "ketosis" can be defined as a state where fat is used to derive energy instead of sugar, thus promoting weight-loss.

However, one thing that should be kept in mind is limiting the number of meals you take per day, or the time span between which you consume food per day, will yield effective results only if you intake less calories than needed.

WHETHER INTERMITTENT FASTING IS SAFE AND HEALTHY?

Usually, intermittent fasting is considered safe to follow, but you must be aware of the risks as well. And above all, before planning for intermittent fasting, you should seek advice from your doctor or physician, especially when the fast is intended to extend for a longer time period.

Following are few cases where intermittent fasting should be avoided as it may result in serious health hazards:

- if you are a diabetic patient

- if you are going through the phase of pregnancy or you are a breastfeeding mother

- if you are taking medications for heart diseases or controlling blood pressure

- if you have issues with disordered eating

- if you have a disturbed sleeping pattern

- if you are too young to try this, like below eighteen years of age

In addition, you should be very careful if you have planned for extended fasting. This means fasting continuously for more than one, two or three days. It is a general precaution that while fasting for period more than 72 hours; you should be kept under strict medical observation.

TIPS FOR INTERMITTENT FASTING

Following are six tips for intermittent fasting that you should follow to maintain healthy weight:

- Drink ample amount of water

- Keep yourself busy

- Include intake of tea or coffee

- Control your hunger waves

- Follow the schedule for at least one month to experience if intermittent fasting promotes healthy weight or not

- Go for a low-carb-diet between periods of fasting. In this way, hunger is reduced, hence making intermittent fasting schedule easy to follow. This not only promotes weight loss but also a reversal of type 2 diabetes.

HOW INTERMITTENT FASTING BENEFITS YOU?

The major benefit of intermittent fasting is weight loss. Nevertheless, there are numerous potential advantages apart from this, few of which are known since ages.

There are different names of fasting periods like "detoxifications", "cleanses" or "purifications", however the concept is same, and that abstains from taking food for a specific time period, usually to gain maximum health benefits. People are of the view that this abstinence period from eating will help in clearing systems in their bodies that deal in eliminating toxins and rejuvenating them. Below are some of the prominent benefits of intermittent fasting:

- Loss of body fat and weight

- Lowering levels of insulin and sugar

- Increase in fat burning

- Possible improvement in concentration and mind clarity

- Possible increase in production of energy

- Possible increase in growth hormone for short time period

- Possible improvement in profile of blood cholesterol

- Possible increase in span of life

- Possible decrease in inflammation

- Possible initiation of cellular cleansing by stimulation of autophagy

- Possible reverse in type 2 diabetes

TECHNIQUES OF INTERMITTENT FASTING

In today's era, intermittent fasting has become a trend among health-conscious individuals. It is claimed that it causes weight loss, improvement in metabolic health, and is also expected to increase lifespan. With the increasing popularity, various methods or techniques of intermittent fasting have been introduced. Each of the methods are highly effective, however, deciding which one gives outstanding results depends on each individual's body system. Following are six popular methods of intermittent fasting.

● The 16/8 Technique: Fasting For Sixteen Hours Everyday

The 16/8 Technique requires you to fast every day for fourteen to sixteen hours and limiting your "eating window" on a daily basis for about 8-10 hours. With your eating window, it is allowed to consume two, three or more meals. Leangains protocol is another name for this technique and was made popular by the fitness guru named "Martin Berkhan".

This technique of fasting is quite simple and is similar to not consuming anything after eating dinner, along with skipping your morning meal. For instance, if you are done with your last meal around 9 pm and avoid eating till 12 pm the next day, this means you observe fast for 15 hours. The important point to note here is that, women are mostly recommended to fast for 14 to 15 hours only, as their body works better if they go for shorter fasts.

If you are among people who feel hungry in the dawn and want to take some food, this method may become quite difficult to follow in the beginning. However, most of the people skipping breakfast are used to this routine and automatically eat this way, without feeling that they have fast for such a long time period.

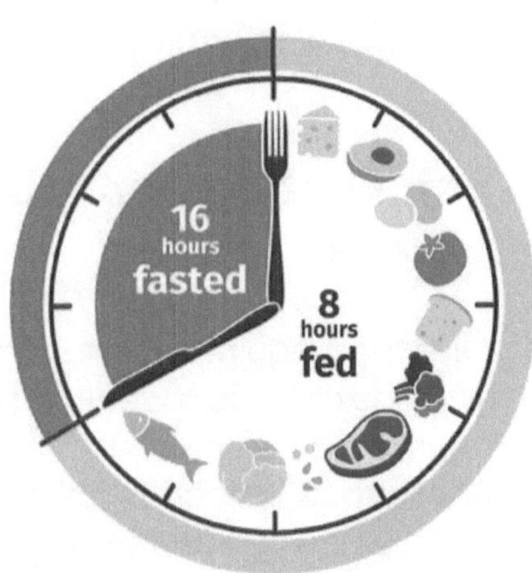

During the fast, you can intake water, coffee and other drinks that do not contribute to increase in calories and also aid in controlling your hunger. You must also realize that it is crucial to consume mainly healthy foods while you have entered into your eating window period. This diet plan will not reveal fruitful results if you keep taking junk foods or high amount of calories.

● The 5:2 Method: Fasting For Two Days Per Week

This type of diet involves consuming food in normal quantity for five days a week while limiting calories within the range of 500 to 600 for 2 days during the week. The 5:2 diet is also known as "The Fast Diet" and was made popular by Michael Mosley, who is a famous journalist of Britain. On the usual days of fasting, it is suggested that women should intake 500 calories while men should take 600 calories. An example in this regard is that you may eat food as usual, all the days of the week except Thursdays and Mondays. For these two days, eating two small portions of meals is enough (i-e, consuming 250 calories in one meal for women, whereas men can have 300 calories per meal). According to critics' point of view, no research has been done to test the 5:2 diet, however there exist numerous studies on the advantages of intermittent fasting.

● Eat-Stop-Eat: Fasting For A Day, Once Or Twice A Week

Eat-Stop-Eat is a diet that requires you to fast for a 24 hour period. You may fast once or twice a week as per your choice. This type of diet was made popular by the health expert named Brad Pilon, and has gained a lot of popularity few years back. In this diet, when you fast from night time on one day to the night time on the next day, this whole period makes 24 hours of fasting.

For instance, you can begin a 24-hour fast by finishing dinner at 8 p.m. Sunday and do not eat till dinner at 8 p.m. the next day. Similarly, you can follow eat-stop-eat diet by fasting from lunch to lunch or breakfast to breakfast, as well. At the end of these efforts, you get the same result. In this diet, coffee, water and other non-caloric drinks are permitted, but solid foods should be avoided during fast. If your primary aim is to shed some weight, it is essential that you consume food normally during the periods when you are allowed to eat. In fact, eat the same quantity of food as when you do not fast at all.

Mo **30**	
Di **31**	
Mi **1**	
Do **2**	
Fr **3**	
Sa **4**	
So **5**	

One of the drawbacks of this diet is that a 24-hour fast often becomes very hard to bear for people. For this reason, you need not start this method right away. You can begin with 14 to 16 hours fasting and then move further. Additionally, you need to self-discipline yourself to complete with the 24-hour fasting so that you do not end up eating before the time limit.

● Fasting On Alternate Days: Fasting Every Other Day

Alternate-day fasting involves fasting every alternate day. You can find numerous different types of this diet plan. Few of these permit around 500 calories while fasting. Several lab studies have shown health benefits gained from intermittent fasting by using few versions of this diet plan. A 24-hour fasting schedule every other day may be considered as an extreme diet plan; therefore it is not suggested for beginners. In this method, you will feel hungry many times and it seems unpleasant as well as unsustainable if you continue it for longer periods.

● The Warrior Diet: Fasting During Day Time, Eating A Big Meal At Night

Ori Hofmekler was the fitness guru who invented The Warrior Diet. This method involves taking food is small portions like raw vegetables and fruits during the day and taking one big meal at dinner. In other words, you fast the whole day, but eat food at night during the four-hour eating window. When you study about the warrior diet, then you find that it is the first diet that includes a type of intermittent fasting and has become popular as well. This type of diet lays emphasis on food choices, which are same as a paleo diet; where eating unprocessed, organic foods are promoted.

● Spontaneous Skipping Of Meals: Skipping Meals Conveniently

In order to reap the fruits of your efforts, you need not follow a well-structured plan for intermittent fasting. Another way to accomplish the ideal weight is skipping meals at times, like when you do not have any feeling of hunger or are quite busy in cooking and eating. It is a bogus concept that you should take food every few hours, otherwise you will go into starvation mode. Our body is such that missing 1 or 2 meals, and handling long periods of starvation is not difficult.

Hence, if you are not very hungry on a certain day, you can omit breakfast and only go for a good lunch and dinner. Likewise, if you are travelling to some place and fail to get anything you wish to eat, you can go for fasting. When you have an inclination towards skipping 1 or 2 meals, it is mainly called "spontaneous intermittent fasting". You should just be careful to consume healthy foods whenever you eat. When you look around yourself, you can find a lot of examples of individuals getting superb results with a few of these techniques. Intermittent fasting is not for every individual and cannot be followed by anyone who wants to lose weight. It is only helpful for some people. For example, intermittent fasting is also not a good option for individuals who have some sort of eating disorders.

WHAT SHOULD YOU INTAKE DURING INTERMITTENT FASTING?

It is a myth that you are allowed to consume anything during intermittent fasting, like highly-processed foods, sugary and fast foods. If your primary aim is to get an ideal weight, increase productivity, and become healthy, you must eat healthy meals. In other words, consuming whole foods, and completely eliminating sugar, carbohydrates and processed foods etc.

Now, it is on you that which type of diet you wish to select, the only condition is that it should be balanced and enhance body fitness. For many people, Keto Diet works as an excellent supplement to diet plans like intermittent fasting since it aids in burning high amount of fat.

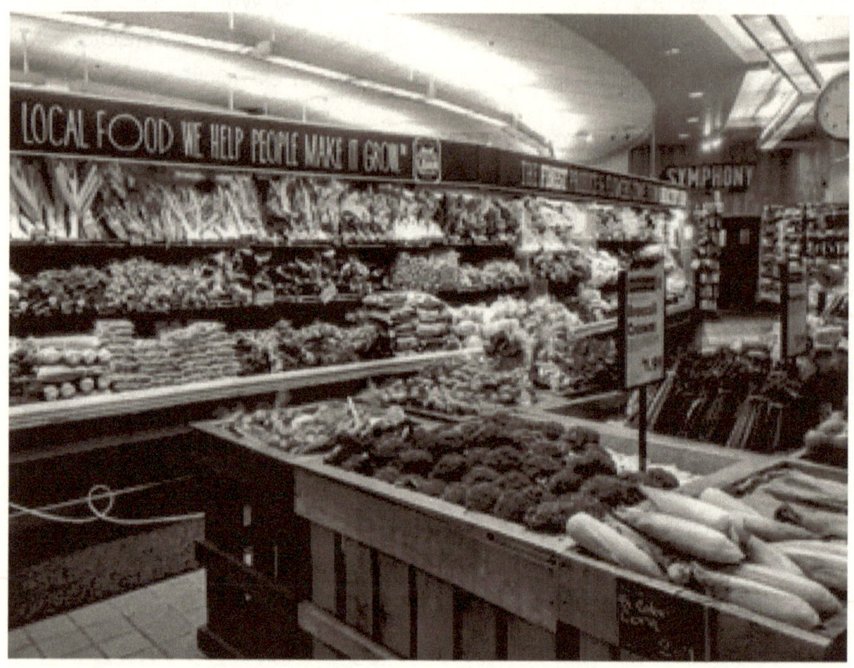

WHAT SHOULD YOU DRINK DURING INTERMITTENT FASTING?

If you are following intermittent fasting, you must strictly avoid taking any caloric food. However, you can take non-caloric drinks as they never break your fast and let you enjoy all the advantages of intermittent fasting, like fat loss, high metabolic rate, decreased level of blood sugar, strong immune system etc. The major reason that non-caloric drinks can be taken is that they do not contribute to release insulin. Therefore, they also have no interference in autophagy and the fat burning process. The non-caloric beverages are as follows:

- Water

- Mineral water

- Sparkling water

- Plain tea

- Plain Coffee

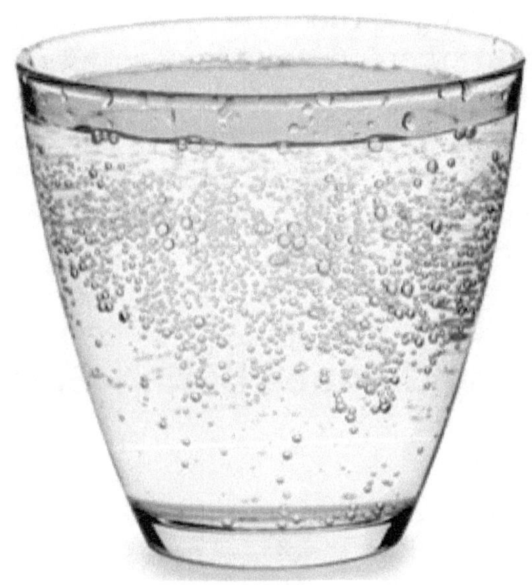

COMMON MISTAKES TO CONSIDER DURING INTERMITTENT FASTING

Many of you face difficulty when following intermittent fasting schedule as you know the real methods, but are unaware of the right approach. That is the reason why an attempt to follow intermittent fasting plan often becomes a failure. Following are few major mistakes that are usually made while fasting:

● An Excuse to Eat Junk Food

Intermittent fasting is an effective way to take control of your eating habits and improve your health. However, you cannot take it as an excuse to eat unhealthy foods believing that intermittent fasting will cancel out the effects of junk food.

When you are fasting, the damaged components in your body are broken down to get energy, while cleaning and healing the body as a whole. Thus, your body responds immediately to the food you consume. If you eat highly nutritious foods, they nourish your body, whereas junk foods do nothing but harm your body. Similarly, your body starts craving for nutrients if you eat junk foods and so, you starve all the time.

● Restricting Calories During 'Eating Window'

When you continue restricting calorie intake even after breaking your fast, you fail to meet the nutrient requirements of your body to perform its functions. Consequently, your overall health is affected adversely. When you take enough food as per your body needs, it releases hormones that give you a feeling of satiety. In this way, your body is fueled to perform the necessary functions.

● Doing a Lot of Things At a Time

Living an unhealthy lifestyle for years does not mean that you start intermittent fasting at once and over-stress your body by following highly strict diet plan. You should start training your body gradually rather than fasting every day, or five days per week or taking low-calorie foods from day 1. These steps can cause major chronic issues in your body.

● Focusing On Time Periods and 'Eating Windows'

Intermittent Fasting fine-tunes your body completely. You learn to follow your body signals indicating feeling of real hunger, and not the clock, where you get ready to eat every 4 hours. Hence, here body becomes the dictator. If you go with the clock for eating, you begin counting down the time and wait anxiously to eat and so, you fail to understand your body signals.

● Low Water Intake

Intermittent fasting helps in detoxification with the help of fluids in your body. Therefore, drinking enough water is essential to eliminate toxins. In fact, increase your water intake more than the usual quantity every day. Water not only keeps you full but also active.

INTERMITTENT FASTING: A COMPLETE GUIDE FOR WEEKLY ROUTINE

You can begin with the journey of Intermittent Fasting easily by following a seven day plan that is not only fun, but also helps you to stick with the target. This plan offers you an action for seven days of the week, with a comprehensive explanation.

● 1ST DAY

TASK: 12 hours Fasting | 12 hour Eating Period

MISSION: Begin with your schedule of Intermittent Fasting

In the beginning, you must move slowly into the schedule of intermittent fasting. Therefore, on the 1st day of the week, you should start with twelve hours of fasting, and then go for sixteen-hour fasting steadily on the 5th day, by fasting one hour additionally each day. In this way, your brain and body become used to of the newly eating plan, as with this technique you offer yourself extensive time to the intermittent fasting. Then, on your 1st day of intermittent fasting, you should also make a choice of the intermittent fasting schedule, which becomes a best fit in your lifestyle. You must always remember that consistency is the key factor that contributes to success.

● 2ND DAY

TASK: 13 hour Fasting | 11 hour Eating Period

MISSION: Learning the basics of IF or Intermittent Fasting

When you are on the 2nd day of the week, you will extend your fast to thirteen hours. This means, you will fast an additional hour than the hours you had fasted yesterday.

On the second day of your fasting, you become acquainted with the rules of healthy eating that aid you in achieving your goals related to Intermittent Fasting. Here, you only need to focus on consuming more amounts of whole foods and eliminating the usual foods that include empty carbs, processed foods, sugars, etc. You can search for simple recipes that are not only delicious but also provide your body essential nutrients. You can go for poached eggs with any vegetable like spinach, meat balls with noodles, salads with different dressings or home-made hummus as a snack.

● 3RD DAY

TASK: 14 hour Fasting | 10 hour Eating Period

MISSION: Decide your rewards

It is essential that when you begin developing a new habit, like intermittent fasting, you must decide about rewards as well. Therefore, on the third day, think about how to reward yourself after every successful fast.

The importance of reward is that it delivers a positive signal to your mind, and encourages you to put more efforts on it. The reward can be anything that makes you contended and happy. The best way in which you can reward yourself for intermittent fasting is considering your needs and planning activities that involve socializing, playing and relaxing. Other types of rewards that are simple but influential are actions of celebrations that are done immediately after achieving the target. These include cheering yourself up while uttering words like "Well done", or highlighting one more day off in your daily progress sheet that you update every day after taking up the challenge. However, if you have decided some bigger reward for yourself, like enjoying dinner at some expensive restaurant, you can opt for token technique. Here, every fasting day allots you one token. When you reach up to five tokens, you give yourself a big treat by going to a restaurant.

● 4TH DAY

TASK: 15 hours Fasting | 9 hour Eating Period

MISSION: Preparing a lunch with high protein content

On the 4rth day of Intermittent Fasting, you observe fifteen hour fasting and as the fast is too long, you should break it with high-protein lunch. This will help in achieving your weight-loss mission. For instance, grilled or steam veggies with any protein you like is a good option. You can take grilled fish, meat, poultry, eggs, tofu, beans, seeds, and nuts, in the form of protein.

● 5TH DAY

TASK: 16 hour Fasting | 8 hour Eating Period

MISSION: Drinking black coffee whenever you get hungry

On the fifth day of Intermittent Fasting week, you are at a point where you will ultimately be reaching your target of 16/8 Intermittent Fasting, that is fasting for sixteen hours and consuming foods during the eight hour window. This goal can be achieved easily if you have patience and follow the guidelines religiously.

In order to aid you in achieving sixteen hour fasting target and curbing your hunger, it is advised to drink black coffee as it is high in antioxidants and also suppresses your appetite. One thing that you should be careful about is that black coffee in intermittent fasting means that no cream, milk, or sugars are added to it. Similarly, flat white or latte, and cappuccino are also not allowed. If you want to give your black coffee a sweet flavor, then you can go for natural sweetener like stevia. If you do not like coffee, then you can take green or black tea, or simply a glass of water as a substitute.

● 6TH DAY

TASK: 16 hour Fasting | 8 hour Eating Period

MISSION: Going for a walk

Apart from controlling you diet, it is also crucial to incorporate some activities in your routine that involve body movement. These activities can be in the form of different exercises like going for a walk before breaking your fast. A twenty minute walk will be very helpful. Walking is an excellent method to enhance your overall health and fitness, and to uplift your mood. When you breathe some fresh air, you feel lively. Walking also aids in switching your concentration from hunger. It enables you to bear those last periods of fasting easily.

● 7TH DAY

TASK: 16 hour Fasting | 8 hour Eating Period

MISSION: Reflecting on your overall progress

On the last day of the 16/8 Intermittent Fasting week, you should review your progress in the past days. This step is important in enjoying fruits of your efforts. What you can do is, capture a full-body picture of your won, measure your weight and then compare these with your photo and weight at the start of the journey. You can see the outcome in the form reduction in both, your weight as well as physical appearance. Additionally, you can ask yourself a few questions to get a clearer picture of your progress. These questions include; how can you describe your feelings, have you noticed some changes in your body energy, skin health, and mood swings from intermittent fasting, and so on. When you carry out this activity, it helps in identifying the reasons for your struggle and where do you actually stand. In this way, you can take action for accelerating your results and incorporating intermittent fasting in your lifestyle.

07

HOW LOW CARB DIET IS HELPFUL TO LOSE WEIGHT?

I congratulate you if you are thinking to go towards a diet that is healthy for your body and that is none other but a low carb diet, also known as ketogenic diet.

● What Is A Low Carb (Keto) Diet?

This diet is not just having low carb foods, but there are so many other things to learn about this diet and the ways to follow it successfully. So basically, first, let's answer that what actually a ketogenic diet is all about? It is a way of eating that include low carb foods that deliver a big quantity of healthy dietary fat and moderate quantities of dietary protein of high-quality.

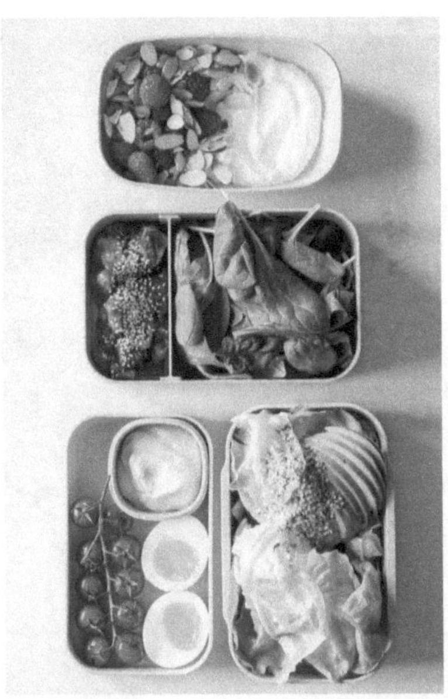

When you reduce the intake of carbohydrate, it shifts your body towards a state that encourages the breakdown of fats (from your body and the diet) for entering ketosis, a state where ketone bodies are produced.

When you follow this type of diet, your whole body, including all the organs and brain rely on ketones as the source of energy. In your body, ketones are produced as you reach a state of ketosis. You can measure whether you are in the state of ketosis through urine and blood tests during the keto diet.

A healthy keto meal is made up of 70 percent of calories coming from fats that are of high-quality, including coconut, seeds, nuts, medium-chain and unsaturated triglyceride oils and avocado, 20 percent of calories from protein, for example grass-fed animal protein and omega-3-rich fish and 10% of it from healthy carbohydrates like berries, legumes, non-starchy vegetables and leafy greens. Here is a chart that shows the percentages of calories provided from fat, protein, and carbohydrate, in a typical ketogenic diet.

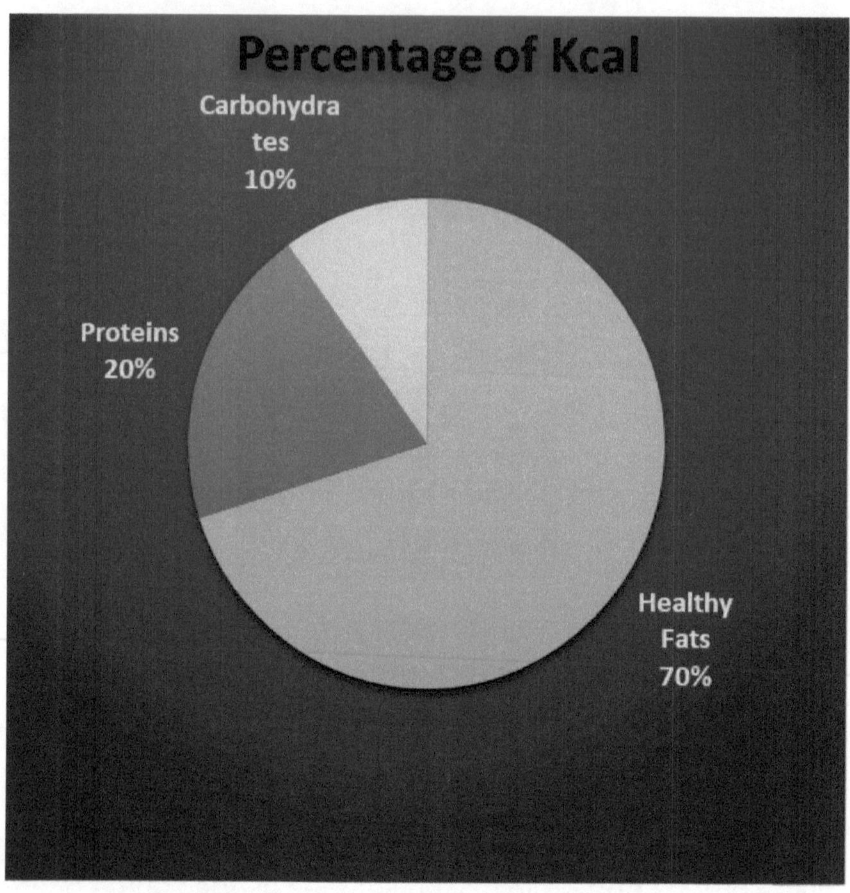

● How It Works?

Our body uses the fuel provided by the food we eat for daily activities, and all the minerals present in the meals help the body grow. For example, a car requires gasoline to keep running, in the same way, our body needs 3 major fuels to keep working, which include proteins, fats and carbohydrates. Carbohydrates are the main element of flour, starch, and sugars which come from plants mostly.

There are two types of fats, which are unsaturated fats, like corn oil that is extracted from plants and saturated fats that come from animals. Then, comes the protein sources such as fish and meat. Other foods come in different variations, for example, nuts which comprises of more than 50% fat.

Protein, fats and carbohydrates, all undergo into a similar chemical reaction with the air we breathe for the purpose of producing energy for the body, and waste products, such as water and carbon dioxide.

This type of similar reaction is also seen when coal or wood are burned or gasoline is burned in a car engine for heat. All of the 3 fuels of the body are also metabolized in the same way. Preferentially, carbohydrates are used, followed by fats and proteins.

The reason why carbohydrates are preferred is because in most people, usually they are readily available, thus, it is easier for the body to metabolize them quickly and produce energy. This is why, athletes are seen eating snacks which contain high carbohydrate prior to an athletic event to have additional energy in their body.

Generally, our body uses carbohydrates within a few hours after their intake, which is why you eat carbs so frequently. The carbs which remain unused are stored in the form of glycogen in the liver, or converted to fat. On the other hand, the main responsibility of fats is to store energy.

Normally, our body stores the fats we eat, however, when there is no sufficient carbohydrate available, the fat stores of the body are broken and used as a fuel. Typically, the metabolism of fats takes place very slowly in a day or so. This is the reason when you have a fatty meal, you feel full as compared to having a low carb meal. Protein, the third fuel, is majorly utilized for building and for refilling body materials; thus any additional protein is excreted or metabolized as fuel. When there is a depletion of fat and carbohydrate stores, the body will start to breakdown muscle for processing the protein for fuel.

The quantity of three fuels in a typical western diet used will be around 60-80% carbs, fats 10-20% and protein 5-15%. The body either stores the additional fuel or excretes it. However, the proportion of fat in the keto diet is increased significantly, whereas the quantity of carbohydrate is reduced greatly. You also need to take care of the total intake of food, as excess food in the body will preferentially discard the fats in an attempt to get back to its desired balance of fuels. The body is pushed to process fats instead of carbohydrates if you limit the total caloric intake.

What actually happens in a keto diet is that it imitates a fasting or starvation state. This is done by not using the carbohydrate the body needs to function normally, instead encouraging metabolism of fat.

As soon this process takes place, ketone bodies are made. The continuous making of the ketone bodies plays a major role to make a ketogenic diet successful. Your body is said to be in ketosis, when it starts to produce ketone bodies. Usually, it takes around 4 to 5 days after starting the diet to enter the state of ketosis.

It is easy to recognize that your body is in ketosis, as the detection of ketones is possible through urine, as well as the change of smell in your breath is also a sign of ketosis. However, it takes several weeks for enjoying the complete effects of a keto diet on your body.

BENEFITS OF A KETOGENIC DIET

Of course, there are a myriad of benefits of starting a keto diet for your health and wellness, some of which include improved cardiovascular health, balanced blood sugar, boost in cognitive performance and weight loss. This is why keto diet is getting popular day by day and many people are opting this lifestyle of having low carbs.

● Weight loss

Several studies show that keto diet also helps in weight management, as it encourages the use of body fat as fuel. Moreover, a ketogenic diet help in reducing cravings and suppressing appetite.

● Management of Blood sugar

There are many research that show low carb diets help in the metabolism of insulin in the body. When there are low or very little carbohydrates, the blood glucose levels are maintained in your body due to breakage of fats and proteins.

● Cognitive ability

When you are on a keto diet, your brain does not use glucose as it major fuel source, rather it uses ketone bodies. Because of this shift, the synaptic connections between brain cells are encouraged which lead to boosted cognitive capabilities, sharper focus and increased mental alertness.

● Metabolic and Cardiovascular health

This diet also supports fatty acid and blood lipid metabolism.

Increased energy

The carbs in your body will go only far to provide energy throughout the day, and specifically during physical activities. However, when your body is in ketosis, it uses fat as fuel rather than glucose, therefore, it provides a consistent supply of the ketone bodies to the brain which is essential to aid workout performance.

● Getting Started

You need to be aware of this fact that when you are following a ketogenic diet, it is important to keep your total carb intake under 50 g a day. So you need to make a lot of changes as compared to the meals you are having currently. The variety of foods present in different sections will help you in planning your snacks and meals so that you can have sufficient amount of fat and protein, while keeping carbohydrates low. You can also take help from your practitioner to get recommendations in each of the following categories for daily servings.

WHAT TO EAT ON A KETO DIET?

Here is a list of some important food categories and quantity that can be take daily in a keto diet.

● Non-starchy Vegetables

- 25 calories (1 serving a day)

- You can have raw leafy green veggies up to 2 to 3 cups

- Other veggies (half cup cooked) (1 cup raw)

- Fat is 0 gram, Protein is 1-2 grams, Carbs is 5 grams

● The non-starchy vegetables may include the following:

- Water chestnuts

- Turnips

- Tomatoes

- Summer Squash (patty pan, crookneck, zucchini, yellow, delicata, spaghetti)

- Snow peas and sugar snap peas

- Sprouts

- Sea Plants nori, kelp, kombu, dulse, arame)

- Sauerkraut

- Rutabaga

- Reddish (watermelon, white icicle, cherry belle, daikon)

- Peppers (sweet, poblano, jalapeno, bell)

- Onions (yellow, green, white, brown, spring, red, shallot, scallions)

- Okra

- Mushrooms

- Lettuce (romaine, red leaf, green leaf, frisee, Boston bibb and butter)

- Leafy greens (watercress , arugula, collard, beet, endive, dandelion, kale, escarole, Swiss chard, spinach, radic-chio)

- Leeks

- Kohlrabi

- Kimchi
- Jicama
- Jerusalem artichoke
- Green or string beans
- Eggplant
- Cucumber
- Bottle gourd
- Celery and Cauliflower
- Asparagus
- String or green beans
- Hearts of palm
- Brussels sprouts
- Bamboo shoots
- Asparagus
- Bitter melon
- Cactus (nopales)
- Cabbage (savoy, red, nappa, green, bok choy)
- Artichoke
- Bean sprouts

DAIRY

- 100 to 150 calories (1 serving a day)

- Fat is 6 to 8 gram, Protein is up to 8 grams, Carbs is 12 grams

● **The dairy may include the following:**

- Whole or full fat milk or plain yogurt (half cup)

- Milk (1 cup)

- Kefir (1 cup, plain)

PROTEIN

- Up to 150 calories (1 serving a day)

- Fat is between 1 to 9 gram, Protein is around 14 to 28 grams, Carbs is 0 grams

● **The protein may include the following:**

- Chicken, dark or white: 3 oz.

- Dark or white Turkey and Venison is 3 oz.

- Goat: 2 oz.

- Shellfish (scallops, shrimp, oysters, crab, mussels, clams, lobster): 4 to 5 oz.

- Bacon: 2 slices

- Feta: 2 oz.

- Elk: 3 oz

- Sausage: varies

- Buffalo: 3 oz

- Eggs, whole: 2

- Herring: 3 oz

- Beef 3 oz (all cuts)

- Skipjack: 4 oz

- Cottage cheese: ¾ cup

- Salmon (Smoked, Fresh or Canned: 3 oz)

- Mackerel: 2 oz

- Egg whites: 1 cup

- Pork, tenderloin, Liver (3 oz.)

- Lamb (lean roast) 3 oz.

- Ricotta: 1/3 cup

- Yellowtail: 4 oz.

- Tuna 4 oz.

- Mozzarella: half cup shredded or 2 oz.

- Trout 4 oz.

- Cornish hen: 4 oz

- Sardines (in oil or water): 3 oz.

FATS AND OIL

- Up to 45 calories (1 serving a day)

- Fat is 5 gram, Protein 0 gram, Carbs is 0 grams

● The fats and oils may include the following:

- 2 table spoon of sour cream

- 1 tsp of sesame oil

- Olives (medium size): 8 to 10

- 1 tsp of extra virgin olive oil

- Half tablespoon of Medium-chain triglyceride powder

- 1 tablespoon of unsweetened mayonnaise

- 1 tsp of sunflower oil

- 1 tsp of safflower oil

- 1 tsp of grapeseed oil

- 1 tsp of butter o ghee

- 1 tsp of flaxseed oil

- 1 tablespoon of cream cheese

- 1 tsp of cream

- 1.5 tsp of coconut spread

- 1 tsp of coconut oil

- 1.5 table spoon of coconut milk (canned, regular) and 3 tablespoon if canned and light

- 1 tsp of canola

- 1 tsp of avocado oil

- 2 tablespoon of Avocado

SEEDS AND NUTS

- Up to 45 calories (1 serving a day)

- Fat is 5 gram, Protein 1 gram, Carbs is 0 grams

● The seeds and nuts may include the following:

- 4 halves of walnuts

- 1 and a half tsp of tahini

- 1 tablespoon of sunflower seeds

- 2 tablespoon of roasted soy nuts

- 1 tablespoon of sesame seeds

- 1 tablespoon of pumpkin seeds

- 12 pistachios

- 1 tablespoon of pine nuts

- 4 halves of pecans

- 3 Macadamia

- 2 tsp of hemp seeds

- 5 hazelnuts

- 1 and a half tablespoon of grounded flaxseed

- 1 and a half tablespoon of shredded and unsweetened coconut

- 1 tablespoon of chia seeds

- 1 and a half tablespoon of cashew butter

- 6 cashews

- 1 and a half tablespoon of almond butter

- 6 almonds

BEVERAGES

The serving for beverages is unlimited.

- Drink filtered water

- Mineral water (carbonated or still)

- Sparkling water (this is the water that is free from artificial flavor and sodium)

- Herbal teas (Non-caffeinated), flavors may include hibiscus, chamomile and mint)

- Unsweetened rooibos tea and green tea

- Espresso (coffee)

SPICES, HERBS AND CONDIMENTS

You can have unlimited servings of Spices, Herbs and Condiments.

- Organic and unsweetened white wine, red wine, Balsamic and apple cider

- Unsweetened tomato sauce

- Dried or fresh spices, such as turmeric, pepper, paprika, onion powder, ginger powder, garlic powder, curry, cumin, cinnamon, cardamom and chili powder)

- Soy sauce, hot sauce

- Blackstrap molasses

- Unsweetened salsa

- Mustard, miso

- Carob

- Liquid amino acid

- Lime and lemon

- Cacao

- Horseradish

- Dried or fresh herbs, including thyme, sage, oregano, mint, rosemary, cilantro, chives, basil and dill

- Ginger and garlic

- Flavored vanilla and almond extracts

- Bone broth

SWEETENERS ALLOWED

It is recommended to take only 1 to2 serving a day, just to decrease craving for sweets.

- Stevia

• **Foods That You Can Occasionally Enjoy**

Legumes (calories = 100) (1 serving)
Fats= 0 to 3 grams, Protein up to 7 grams and Carbs = 15 grams
• Half cup of cooked Peas
• French, yellow, red, green or brown lentils
• 4 tablespoons of hummus
• ¾ cup of homemade bean soup
• Half cup of refried vegetarian beans
• Half cup of cooked beans including pinto, navy, mung, lima, kidney, garbanzo, edamame, cannellini and black eyed

Berries (calories = 60) (1 serving)
Fats= 0 grams, Protein= 0 grams and Carbs = 15 grams
1¼ cup of strawberries
One cup of Raspberries
¾ cup of Loganberries
Half cup of unsweetened cranberries
¾ cup of boysenberries
¾ cup of blueberries and blackberries

FOODS YOU HAVE TO AVOID

FOODS	EXAMPLES
Fast Foods	Pasta Burger And Pizza
Foods That Claim That Are Sugar Free, But Contain Artificial Sweeteners	Sucralose, Acesulfame K And Aspartame (Diet Cokes)
Alcoholic Sugar Drinks	Cocktails And Sweet Wines
Fats (Unhealthy)	Vegetable Oils (Processed)
Tubers And Root Vegetables	Carrots And Potatoes
Fruits	All, Except Restricted Quantity Of Berries Are Allowed
Wheat Based Products, Starches Or Grains	Cereal, Pasta And Rice
Sauces And Processed Sugary Foods	Candies, Ice Creams, Smoothies, Fruit Juices And Soda

KETOSIS

The state in which the body fat is broken down for energy by the liver is known as ketosis. During this process, ketone bodies are produced, which are of 3 types.

- beta-hydroxybuterate acid

- acetoacetate

- acetone

As we enter the state of ketosis, our body starts to spill the ketone acetoacetate. Thus, a small part converts into the ketones acetone spontaneously and then changes into beta-hydroxybuterate enzymatically. Beta-hydroxybuterate is used by the brain as a source of energy.

During this duration, most of the people complain of bad breath, however, this is from acetone and completely normal and it goes away with time.

Most of the cells in your body can directly utilize these ketones for energy, just as they do for glucose. Still, some cells require glucose, such as the cells in your eyes and red blood cells. However, you do not need to worry, as your liver already possess a glucose generator. This generator helps in producing glucose from protein. This procedure is also known as gluconeogenesis. Thus, your liver has the ability to make sufficient sugar necessary for those vital cells to use.

- Ketoadcidosis

When it comes to ketosis, the biggest fear that health care experts have is the chances of it going too far, into a condition, known as ketoacidosis. During this state, the level of your ketones becomes very high, thus converting your blood very acidic.

However, if your pancreas are working fine, then you do fall into this risk, but people with type 1 diabetes are likely to get into this state of Ketoadcidosis, thus, it is important for people with Type 1 diabetes to take recommendation for a health-care professional before they start a keto diet.

You are safe to start a keto diet if:

- You have pre-diabetes

- Not taking insulin but have a type-2 diabetes

- Have a metabolic syndrome

WAYS TO REACH THE STATE OF KETOSIS

It is pretty easy to achieve ketosis, however, it seems confusing and complicated for people because of excess of information present on the internet. In simple and easy word, here is what you need to do in levels of significance to reach ketosis:

● Limiting Your Carbs

You do not need to just concentrate on net carbs, rather, it is essential to control your daily intake of carbs for best results. You have to limit under 35grams of carbs per day and below 20g net carbs.

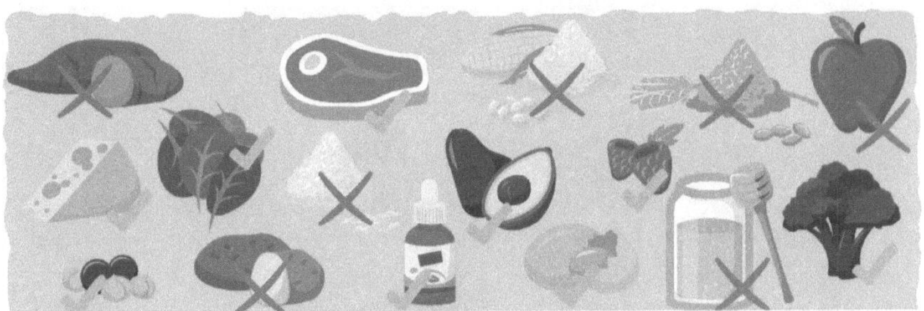

● Limiting Your Intake Of Protein

Always remember to take a moderate amount of protein as having too much quantity of protein may result in lower levels of ketosis. Eat around 0.5 to 0.8 grams of protein per pound of your body mass if you want to lose weight successfully. You can also take the help of a keto calculate for easier calculations.

● Do Not Take the Stress Of Eating Fats

During keto, the major source of energy is Fat. Therefore, ensure you are having sufficient amount of fat in your diet. The keto diet does not endorse starvation for weight loss.

● Hydrate Yourself

It is ideal to drink at least one gallon of water a day. It is important to have plenty of water and also stay consistent with the quantity of water you drink. This helps in controlling your hunger levels as well as helps in the regulation of several vital bodily functions.

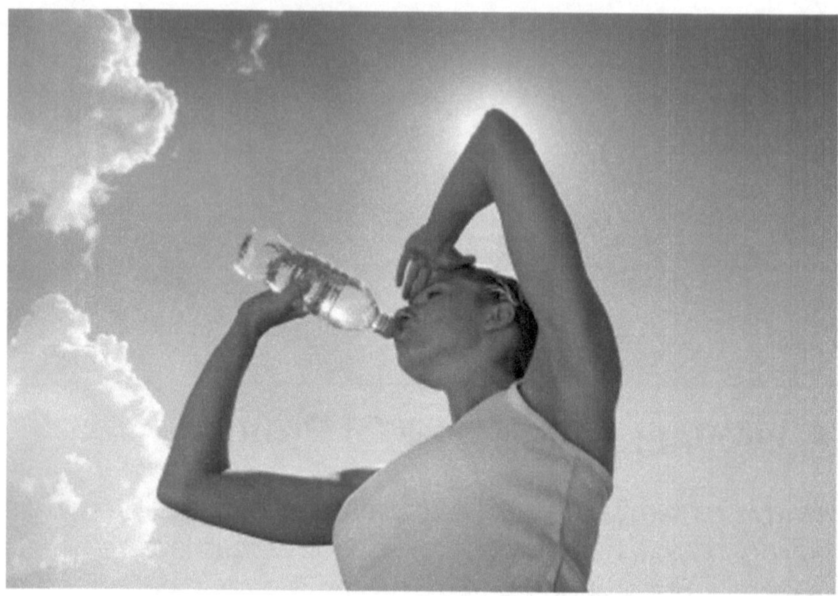

● Do Not Eat Unhealthy Snacks

You can achieve your ideal weight when you have fewer insulin spikes during the day. Eating snacks unnecessarily will make your weight loss process slower.

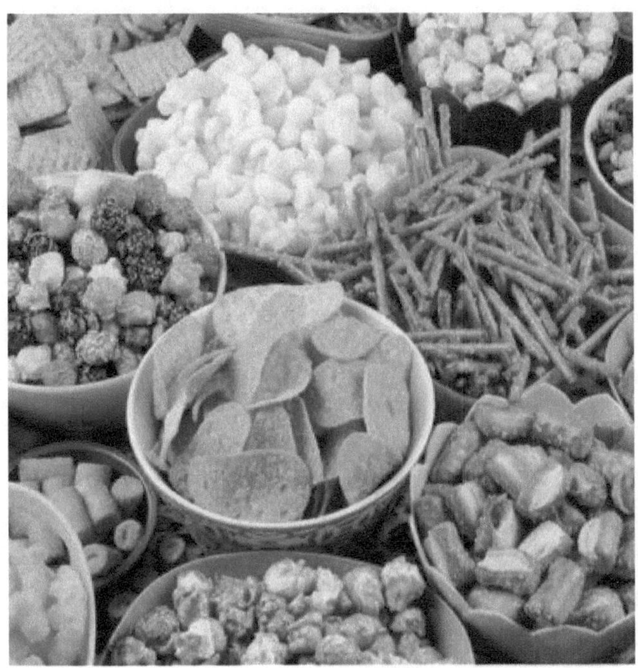

● Make Fasting A Part Of Your Lifestyle

You can consistently boost our ketone levels through fasting. There are several methods of fasting that you can read about in other chapters.

● Add Exercise In Your Routine

The significance of exercise is undeniable. Consider doing 15 to 30 minutes of daily exercise if you want to get the most out of your low carb diet. If you are not into high intensity exercise, then try low intensity physical activities, for example, just walk for a few minutes help in the regulation of blood sugar levels and weight loss.

HOW TO FIND OUT THAT YOU'RE IN KETOSIS?

When you are in the state of ketosis, your body does not depend on carbs anymore for energy, rather it prefers burning of fat for fuel. Once you increase dietary fat and limit the intake of carbohydrates, ketone bodies are formed due to fat metabolism.

There are a number of methods to monitor Ketones. These include the following.

- **URINE STRIPS:** A very common method to check for ketosis is using a urine testing strip. The color of the strip changes according to the presence of acetoacetate in urine. However, with this method, you cannot match ketone levels present in the blood due to some factors, especially water intake, which may lead to a false positive with over-hydration or dehydration. With time, when your body is able to use ketone bodies as fuel, this result in decreased excretion of ketones, which results in false negative readings when you use urine strips for testing of ketosis.

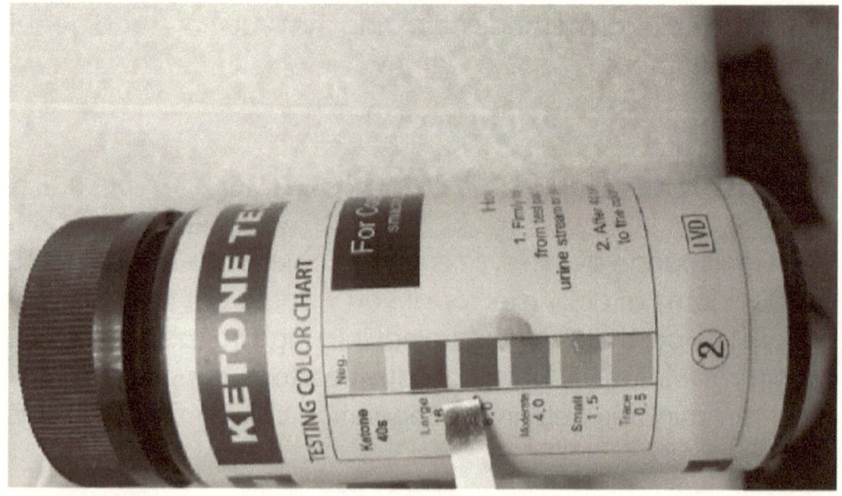

- **BREATH METER:** Beta-hydroxybutyrate is the main ketone body present in your blood. As it gets metabolized, it is converted into acetoacetate and afterwards acetone. You can measure these changes using a breath meter device.

- **BLOOD METER:** Another effective method for the measurement of the levels of ketones is blood meter. But this method is costly as compared to other and also more invasive. You can take advice from your healthcare practitioner on using the most suitable blood meter for testing ketone levels.

Besides testing, there are also many physical symptoms that indicate if you have reached ketosis. These include the following.

- **INCREASED ENERGY AND REDUCED HUNGER:** When you have reached an optimal level of ketones in your body, you'll experience an energized or clear mental state and a much lower hunger level.

- **BAD BREATH:** A ketone body, known as Acetone is excreted in your breath. The smell of Acetone is like a nail polish remover or an over ripe fruit. However, it goes away with time.

- **INCREASE IN URINATION AND DRY MOUTH:** Another symptom of ketosis is increased urination, which results in increased thirst and dry mouth. Thus, make sure to replenish your electrolytes (magnesium, potassium and salt) by drinking sufficient water.

COMBINING KETO DIET WITH INTERMITTENT FASTING

The eating regime of the keto diet includes moderate protein, low carb and high fat. This trains your body to consume fat as a major fuel. You need to start keto diet to begin this process, as the body utilizes glycogen stores quickly when you eat low carb meals. In this way, you immediately enter into ketosis. Generally, this starts within 2 to 3 days.

The next shift takes place when your body starts burning fat for fuel. This takes around 3 to 6 weeks. Finally, you are fat adapted and whenever you are fasting, your body starts using your fat reserves automatically. This is one of the major advantages of combining keto and intermittent fasting.

It becomes difficult to stick with fasting and eating plan if you lack the motivation. So the question arises how to keep your morals high? Here are some of the important reasons that will help you to achieve your goals while you enjoy the necessary incentives along the way. When keto diet and fasting are done together, it provides following benefits for your health.

- Increased energy

- Increased focus

- Autophagy (the process in which old cells are broken and recycled by the body)

- Heart health (reduced blood pressure and cholesterol levels)

- Weight loss

- Decreased inflammation linked with several chronic illnesses

- Reduced levels of insulin

SUPPLEMENTING YOUR KETO DIET

Even though you have to eat low carb foods during a keto diet, but there are many ways of supplementation to benefit your diet using different ketogenic products. You can take advice from your healthcare practitioner regarding the incorporation of these products into your daily diet plan. Some of these products include the following:

- **EXOGENOUS KETONE SALTS:** Have keto salts in your diet as it helps in increasing the circulation of ketones in your body, which can be used as an additional source of energy afterwards.

- **KETOGENIC SOUPS AND SHAKE:** Another way to supplement your keto diet is to have keto soups and shakes. They are an ideal pre-/postworkout snack and a meal replacement as these are easy to make and provides a great support for a keto lifestyle.

- **MCT POWDER AND MCT:** Make sure to add medium-chain triglycerides (MCT) of high quality in your ketogenic lifestyle to make the most of your diet. These are available in both oil and powder forms and can be easily added to shakes and meals. The MCT powder and oil are 90% concentrated of C10 and C8 fatty acids, as well as provide 10 grams of MCT in every serving.

HOW TO MAINTAIN KETOSIS?

It may be possible that you are following the keto diet and also fasting along with it for a few weeks but still not shedding any pounds. This question may come in your mind that where am I doing wrong? It becomes frustrating when you don't achieve your target results and this can make you want to give up. So here I am listing down some of the possible reasons that why you are not losing weight even after following the diet.

● You Have Not Reached Ketosis

As you start to follow this diet, you may assume that you have reached the state of ketosis, but that is always not true. The possibility is you are calculating or recording your intake of calories incorrectly. Therefore, it is recommended to check whether you have reached ketosis through urine strips. You can also find this out using a ketone breath analyzer, or get a blood ketone monitor for accurate results.

● Eating Too Many Carbs

As you are new to intermittent fasting and keto diet, you should remember the most important aspect of this diet and that is you have to take care of your intake of carbs. Even though you are taking low carb veggies, it may be possible that there are hidden sugars that is hampering your weight loss.

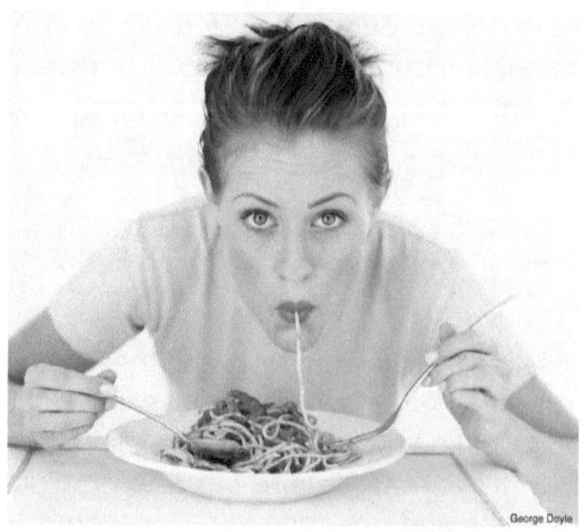

Find out whether you are consuming products that are sugar free? If yes, then these products may contain hidden sugars, such as xylitol and sorbitol that you are consuming without knowing their effects on your diet. Most of the substitutes of sugar cause higher insulin levels which delays your weight loss. Besides, avoid store bought condiments and salad dressings as they consist of a lot of carbs.

Instead, have keto friendly versions of condiments, or make your own keto spices, such as homemade mayonnaise is generally used in every salad dressing. Look for the culprit that's postponing your progress to achieve your weight loss target.

● Eating Excessively

Though you have controlled your intake of carbohydrates, it does not mean you can overeat other group of foods. This is because when you eat more calories than required, you can easily gain weight. Be mindful that you also need to recheck the amount of calories you are taking through fats and as you start losing weight, the requirement of calories that your body needs also reduced. It is wise to recheck your counts and to keep track of that info after every 5 pounds you lose. There are several food tracker apps available on the internet, which can help you in this regard.

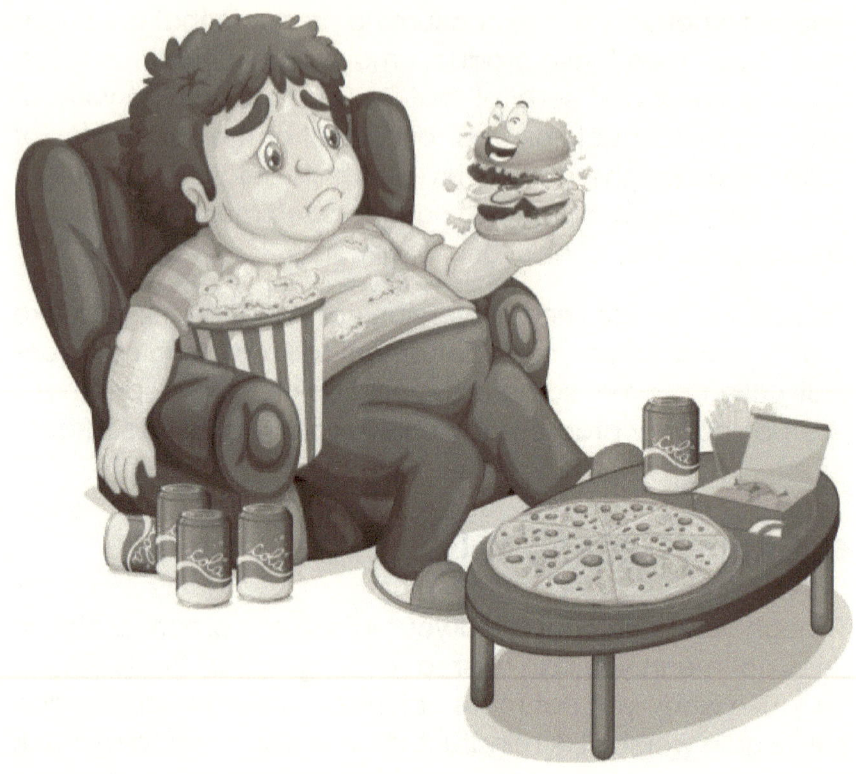

● Eating Excessive Amount of Protein

If you see that in spite of all efforts, you are not losing weight, you may need to recalculate your protein needs. This is because if you eat lots of protein, it leads to gluconeogenesis. This is a procedure that transforms protein into sugar. Moreover, do not have liquid protein, especially drinks or shakes as they easily change into sugar.

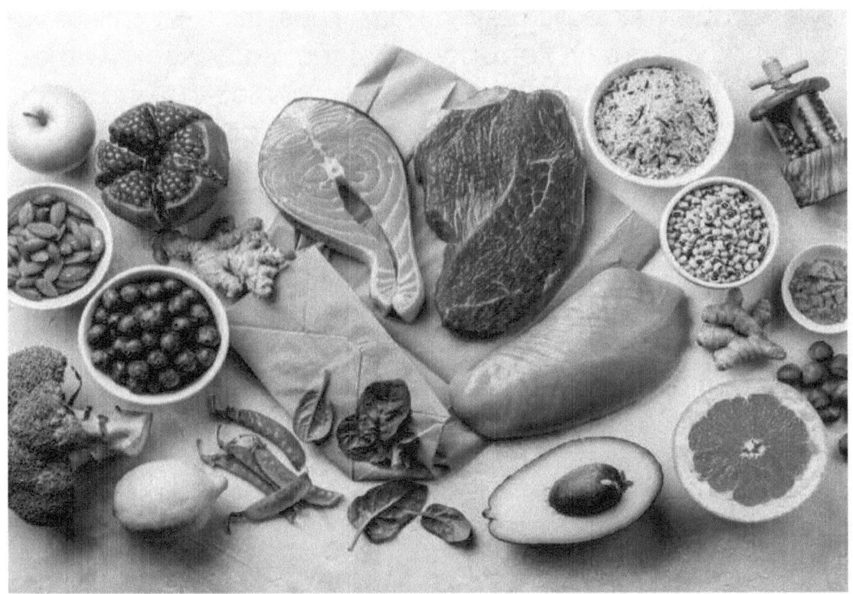

● You Are Not Fasting In a Proper Manner

Go for a more restrictive and longer fast instead of a 16:8, if you see you are not getting results. You can begin with an alternate day fast once a week and then increase its frequency up to 2 to 3 times in 7 days. This type of fasting is considered as the best fasting for quick weight loss and when you combine it with the keto diet, you will feel much less hunger.

● You Are Fasting All the Time

You shouldn't be fasting daily or back to back every alternate day as doing so can mess up with your metabolism. It is important to take breaks while fasting, for example, break of 1 week, after every 3 weeks of fasting for resetting your metabolism. This won't be an issue for you if you're new to intermittent fasting and keto. Just remember, when you fast all the time, it lowers your metabolism eventually. Thus, to avoid this situation while you are on keto, don't fast too many weeks without a break or back to back days. By following all the above tips, you can prevent a plateau on intermittent fasting and keto.

For a successful lifestyle, planning is one of the major attributes. Intermittent fasting and keto are no different. It is necessary to find the times that are right for you to fast if you successfully want to achieve your target weight. Sticking to that plan of taking keto snacks and meals are important. Besides, it is essential for you to learn how intermittent fasting works and the basics of the ketogenic diet in order to be successful in this journey.

USEFUL TIPS TO FOLLOW KETO DIET SUCCESSFULLY

The step towards following intermittent fasting and keto diet together surely leads you to a healthy lifestyle. This not only helps you in losing weight but also improves your health. Below mentioned are a few useful tips that enable you to follow a keto diet successfully and enjoy fruitful results:

● Tracking Your Food

You can find numerous apps that allow you to keep track of the amount of carbs and calorie consumption, and any other thing you want to have a record of. When you become aware of what and how much you are eating, you can actually point out your mistakes and where you need to improve. Hence, a keto diet app is quite useful for this purpose.

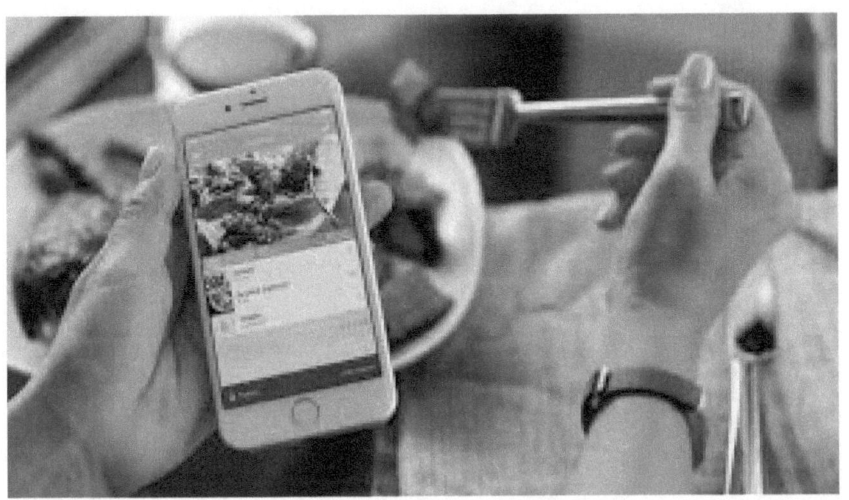

● Finding a Community

To adopt a new lifestyle is definitely a daunting task. It is crucial that you should have some support in the form of friends or closed ones with whom you can discuss your issues, queries and fears. If you do not have a better-half or a friend who is a partner in your diet plan, you need not worry since there a number of online communities that increase your motivation and understand you in times of need.

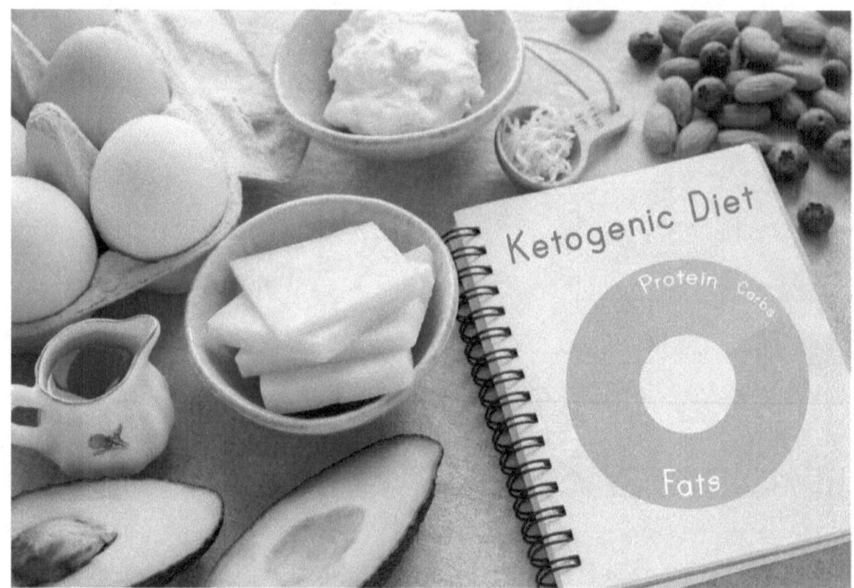

● Never Lose Hope

When you begin with the fasting and keto diet, you may experience a quick reduction in your weight, but it may later stop on a certain figure. At that time, you may start thinking that keto diet is not working anymore and give up. You should consider the fact that you gained weight over a period of time and so it will take some time to lose weight as well. It is a time taking process and you must have patience to get good results.

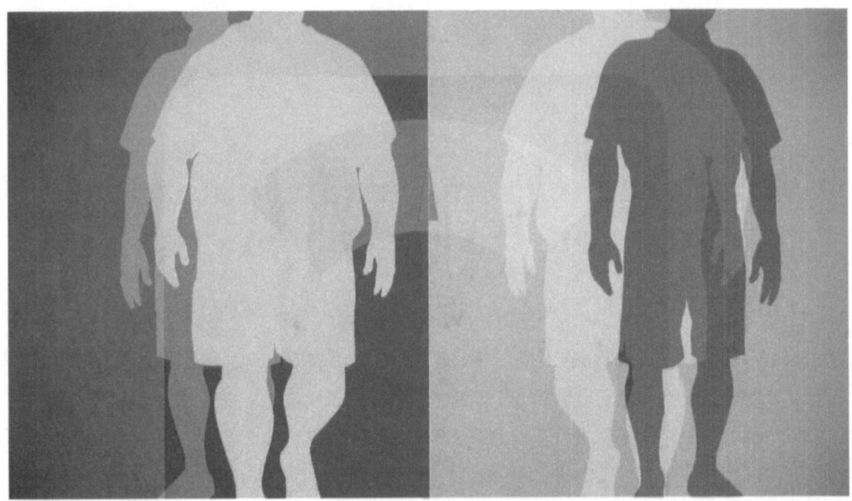

If you follow the rules of ketogenic diet and intermittent fasting religiously, you can get amazing results concerning your physique and overall health. When you plan your meals and adhere to a schedule, it keeps you motivated and your belly remains full. If you feel lonely and need companionship in your weight-loss journey, you can connect with supporting communities to get the guidance.

FREQUENTLY ASKED QUESTION CONCERNING KETO DIET

- ## How can you define keto-adaptation? How much time is needed to adapt?

The process in which your body experiences changes during the keto diet plan, and uses fat as a source of energy instead of glucose, it is called Keto-adaptation. The time required for adaptation varies for every individual, however usually it begins within a few days, soon after you go on a keto diet. After seven to fourteen days, you can see positive results of keto-adaptation on your body.

● What visible changes can you expect from the keto-adaptation process?

When you follow the keto-adaptation process, you may experience a few minor effects known as the "keto flu." Such changes take place when your body undergoes the process of moving towards burning fat rather than carbohydrates as the principal energy source. You may feel drowsiness, dizziness, nausea, and body aches during this process. Other changes that you can experience include stomach pains, muscle soreness and cramping.

● When these effects are going to end?

Mostly keto flu lasts for less than or maximum seven days for an average individual, however, again you must understand that not everybody experiences such effects. Following are a few techniques that you can use to aid your body through this keto flu:

- Increasing electrolyte intake, while avoiding electrolyte drinks containing high sugar content.

- Drinking a lot of water

- Eating high quantity of quality fat

- Taking an exogenous supplement of ketone salt

- Doing regular exercise

- Maintaining your sleeping schedule

● How long can the ketogenic diet be continued? Is there any harm if you continue for a longer time period?

It purely depends on your target that how long ketogenic diet can be continued. Your health advisor may suggest a certain time period for which you can follow keto diet. You will find several people that take ketosis as a challenge and stick with it for an extended time period without experiencing any adverse effects.

● Can ketogenic diet alter your cholesterol levels and raise it further?

If you intake high cholesterol foods, it creates a little effect on your cholesterol levels in your body. In fact, triglycerides in your blood are the main risk factors for your cardiac diseases and are directly connected to the carbohydrates in your diet. When you follow a low-carb diet, it decreases serum triglyceride levels tremendously. Your health advisor may keep a check on your cholesterol levels to make sure that they do not cross the normal range while following the keto diet.

● What amount of weight is expected to lose with keto diet?

It depends on you that how much you want to lose weight. If you include regular workouts in your schedule, it will accelerate your weight-loss process. Likewise, eliminating certain foods that directly contribute in weight gain also helps a lot. These include; dairy, artificial sweeteners, wheat products and its by-products like; wheat flours, wheat gluten etc.

Weight loss through water consumption is also quite common if you begin with the low-carb diet. With Ketosis and water intake, you may experience a diuretic effect on your body that may result in weight loss within a few days. This is a prominent sign that your body has now become accustomed to adjusting itself as a machine that promotes fat burning process.

● How can you keep track of your carbohydrate intake?

You can keep track of your carbs through various apps. The best among them is MyFitnessPal. You will not be able to track net carbohydrates taken on this app, but you can calculate total carbohydrates taken by you along with the total fiber. In order to calculate net carbohydrates, total fiber consumed is subtracted from total carbohydrates consumed.

● What if you cheat and then wish to carry on with keto diet? How can you do it?

If you have cheated for some time and now wish to go back to the ketogenic diet again, then there are no issues. For the time being your weight increases since your body has the ability to retain water. Again, the weight falls down quickly as soon as the water is lost. If you see that the scale fluctuates easily, then do consider the fact that there exists a biological reason for the change. What you need to do is, motivate yourself, get back on your keto schedule and stick to it strictly while controlling your cravings.

● What to do if you fail to lose any weight further?

There are several factors that decelerate the process of weight loss like lack of sleep, depression, stress, hormonal changes, exercise, and use of alcohol and so on. Weight loss has never been a linear process. The weight scale fluctuates readily everyday due to water changes.

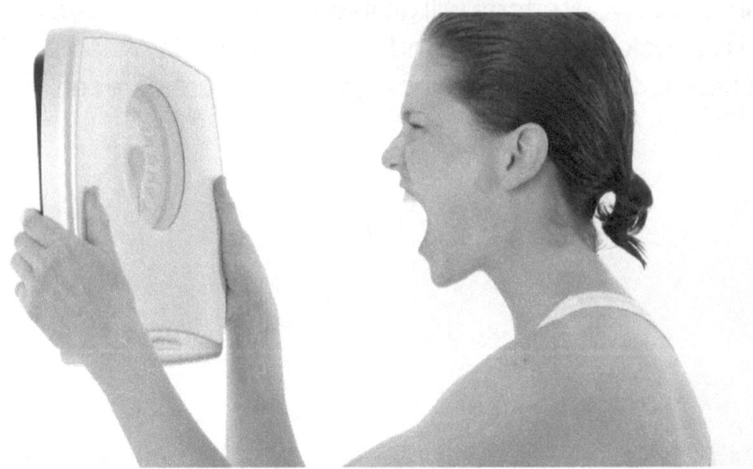

An individual loses weight around one to two pounds on average per week; however this does not reflect that the weight scale will fall consistently. You should not only measure weight through scale but also take body measurements, as it may happen that there are changes in body size but no alterations on the scale. What you should do is drink lots of water and supplement electrolytes. Additionally, reduce the quantity of dairy from your diet.

● What to do once you attain your goal weight through keto?

There are individuals who want to go off with the ketogenic diet after reaching their target weight, whereas others continue with the diet or change their life style by adopting clean-eating. One thing that you should never forget is that if you go back to junk foods and unhealthy eating, you will gain weight again and all your efforts will go in vain. You must always try to keep a check on your diet, and avoid junk foods. You may still experience gain in weight since glycogen stores are refilled.

KETO FRIENDLY RECIPES

Here are some amazing keto friendly recipes, including breakfast, lunch, dinner, snacks, drinks and dessert. You can try these delicious, yet healthy recipes while you are on a keto diet.

1. CHORIZO KETO OMELETTE

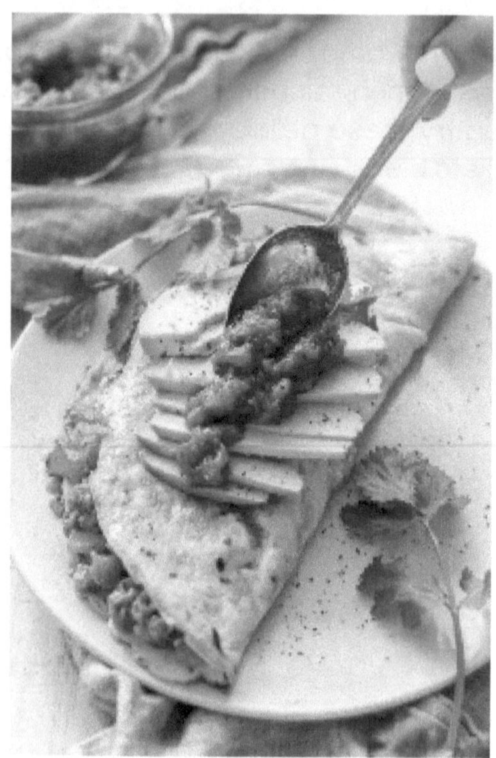

INGREDIENTS

For Omelette

- Heavy Whipping Cream 2 tablespoons

- Eggs - 2 Large

- Salt & Pepper (as per your taste)

- Spinach, 1/4 Cup (Chopped)

- Cheddar Cheese (1/4 Cup) - Shredded

- Chorizo – 2 ounces

- White Onion 2 Tablespoons

Toppings

- Sour Cream - 1 Tablespoon

- Avocado - 1/8 cup (diced)

- Bacon - 1 Slice (Crumbled)

DIRECTIONS

- First of all, you have to cook Chorizo as per the instructions mentioned on the packet.

- Now whisk onion, whipping cream, spinach and eggs in a medium bowl.

- Take a non-stick skillet and pour this mixture and put it at low to medium heat

- When omellete is firm enough, then flip it.

- Cook evenly, while you sprinkle Cheese on the other side of the omellete.

- Once it is done, take it and place on plate

- The next step is to roll the egg after adding Chorizo to omelette.

- Top it with Bacon, Chorizo, Diced Avocado and Sour Cream.

2. KETO CHEESE SANDWICH

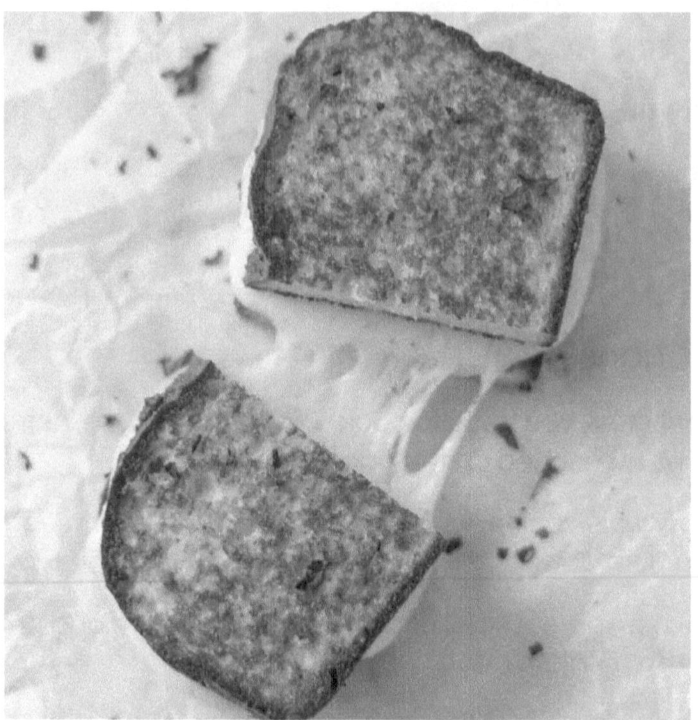

INGREDIENTS

- Pepper and salt according to taste

- sausage patties – 2

- Sriracha – half tsp

- Avocado – ¼ (sliced) (medium)

- Cheddar – 2 tbsp

- Cream cheese – 1 tbsp

DIRECTIONS

- Cook sausages over medium heat in a skillet according to the directions given on the packet.

- Place cream cheese in small bowl and sharp cheddar. After this, microwave it for a half minute until melted

- Now, mix sriracha with cheese, set aside

- The next step is to mix egg with all the seasoning and fry a small omelette

- Finally, use the mixture of sriracha and cheese to fill the omelette and assemble sandwich.

3. SCRAMBLED EGGS WITH SMOKED SALMON AND SPINACH

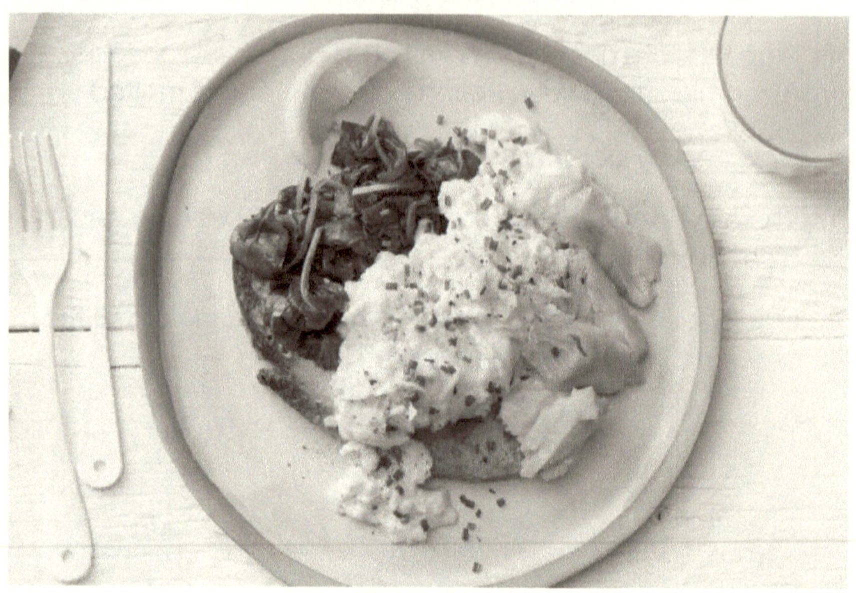

INGREDIENTS

- Cooked Bacon Or Smoked Salmon - 1 Oz.

- Heavy Whipping Cream - 2 Tbsp

- Butter - 1 Tbsp

- Ground Black Pepper And Salt (As Per Your Taste)

- Eggs - 2

- Baby Spinach - 1 Oz

DIRECTIONS

- Take a fry pan and heat the butter. Add the baby spinach and fry until soft.

- Now the next step is to add the cream in the fry pan. Let it cook for a few minutes until you see a creamy texture.

- After this, put eggs in the pan and stir it properly. After this, season it with pepper and salt. Keep on stirring the mixture until it's cooked. Finally, take a plate and put the scrambled eggs on it and serve together with smoked bacon or salmon.

4. KETO POPPER JALAPENO CHAFFLES

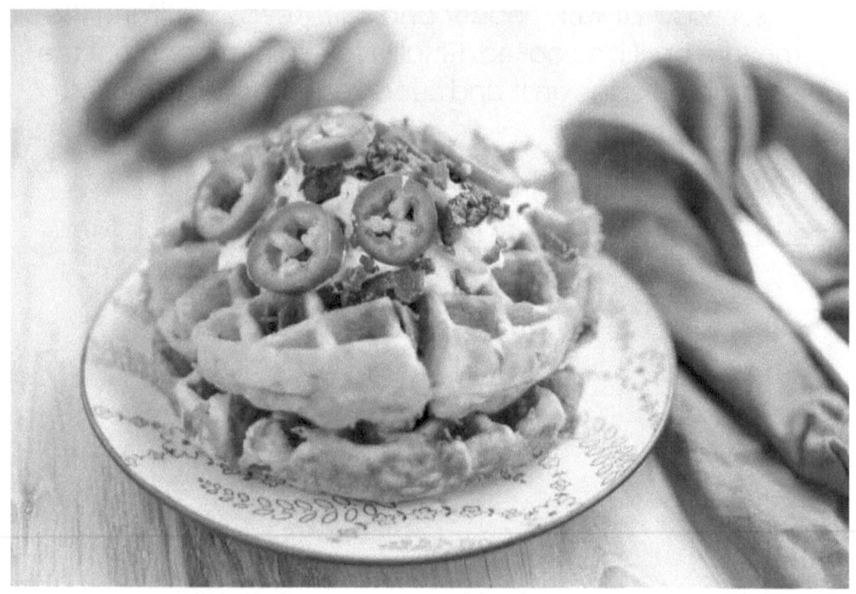

INGREDIENTS

For Chaffles:

- Fresh And Chopped Chives - 2 Tbsp

- Cheddar Cheese - 8 Oz (Shredded)

- Eggs - 4

For Topping

- Cream Cheese - ½ Cup (Softened)

- Scallion - 1 (Chop It Finely)

- Garlic Cloves - ½ Tsp (Minced)

- Jalapeños - 2 Fresh (Sliced And Seeded)

- Bacon - ½ Cup (Cook And Chop It)

DIRECTIONS

- First of all, take the waffle maker and pre-heat it.

- Take a bowl and place all the ingredients and mix it.

- Now grease your waffle iron slightly and then put the mixture evenly over the bottom plate.

- Cook for around 5 minutes after closing the waffle iron.

- As soon as it is done, lift the lid gently.

- Place the spring onions, garlic and cream cheese into a bowl while the waffles cook and beat well to combine.

- The next step is to ass most of the bacon, leave some for garnishing.

- As the waffles are cooked, top it with chopped bacon, chives, sliced jalapeno and cream cheese.

1. GREEN SALAD WITH SMOKED SALMON AND AVOCADO

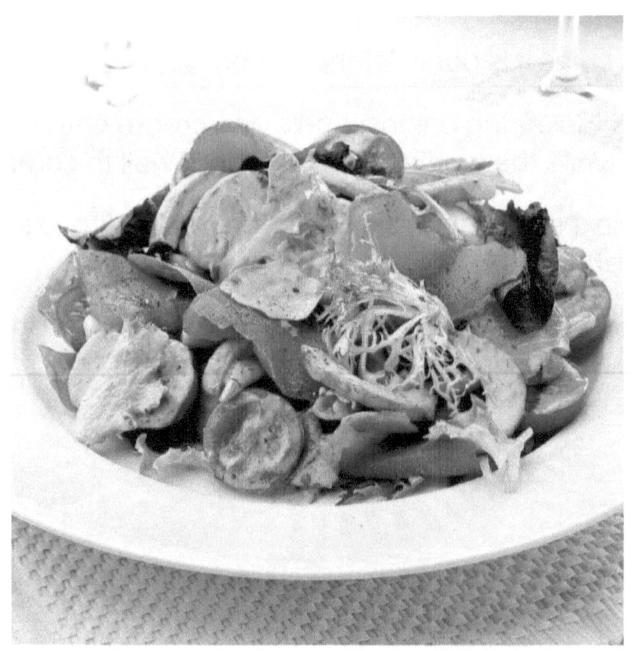

INGREDIENTS

- Egg – 1

- Extra Virgin Olive Oil – 1 tablespoon

- Mixed Greens - 1 ½ cup

- Sea Salt & Black Pepper (to taste) – 1/8 tsp

- Avocado (sliced) – 1/4

- Smoked Salmon – 50 grams

DIRECTIONS

- Hard boil the eggs by placing them in a small pot of boiling water. Cook for 7 minutes (or to your liking), and when done, transfer to a bowl of ice water to cool. Once cool, peel and slice into halves.

- Divide the greens into bowls and add the olive oil and salt. Toss gently to mix well, then place the avocado on top, as well as the eggs and the salmon. Enjoy!

2. FRIED HALLOUMI WITH CUCUMBER AND AVOCADO

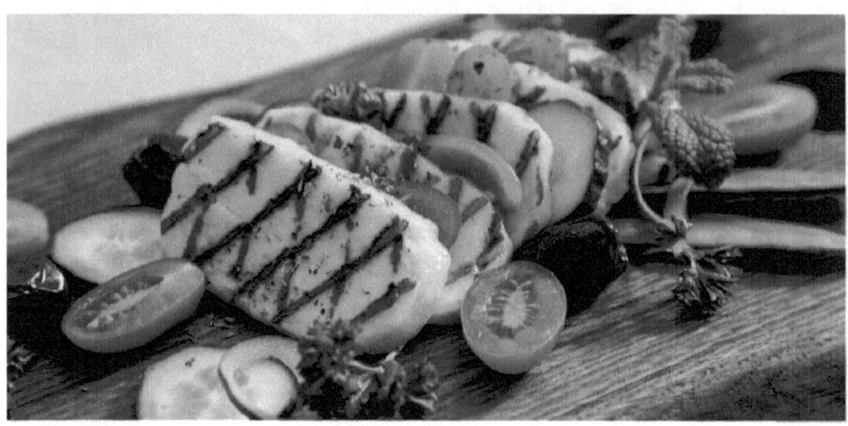

INGREDIENTS

- Avocado Oil (divided) – 1 tablespoon

- Halloumi (halved, patted dry) Avocado (pit removed, halved) – 160 grams

- Cucumber (sliced) – ½

- Cherry Tomatoes (halved) - ½ cup

- Sea Salt & Black Pepper (to taste) – 1/8 tsp

- Black Olives (pitted) – ¼ cup

DIRECTIONS

- Heat the oil in a pan over medium to high heat. Add the halloumi slices to the pan and cook until browned; about 1 to 2 minutes per side.

- Divide the halloumi, avocado, tomato, olives, and cucumber onto plates. Season with salt and pepper. Enjoy

3. ZUCCHINI ALFREDO WITH TURMERIC CHICKEN

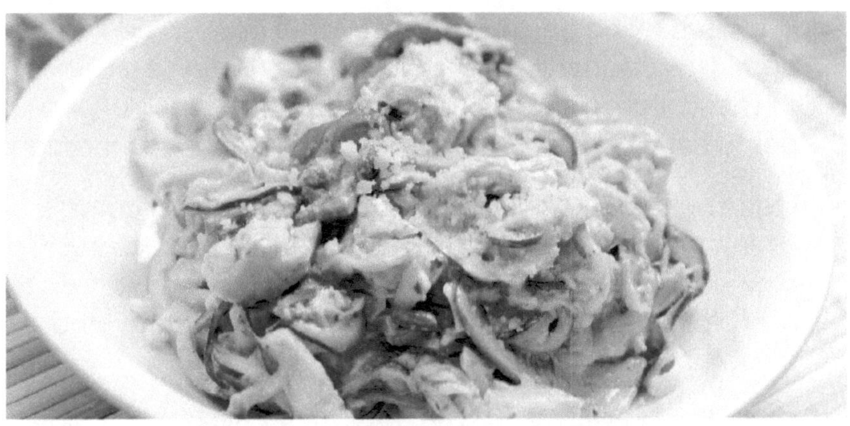

INGREDIENTS

- Zucchini – 2

- Turmeric – 1 tsp

- Sea Salt & Black Pepper (a pinch to taste) -1/4 tsp

- Lemon juice – ½

- Plain Coconut Milk – 1 cup

- Avocado (peeled and pit removed) – 1 ½

- Italian seasoning 1 tsp

- Chicken Breast (sliced) – 230 grams

- Coconut Oil – 1 tablespoon

DIRECTIONS:

Spiralize the zucchini or use a julienne peeler to create noodles. Set aside.

- In a large frying pan, heat the coconut oil over medium heat. Then, add the chicken to the pan. Sprinkle it with turmeric, Italian seasoning, sea salt, and a pinch of pepper to taste. Saute for 10 minutes, or until cooked through.

- Meanwhile, make the avocado cream sauce by combining the avocado, coconut milk, and lemon juice in a blender or food processor. Add a pinch of sea salt and black pepper to taste, and blend until creamy and smooth.

- Once the chicken is cooked through, transfer it to a plate. Now, add the zucchini noodles back into the pan and saute the zucchini noodles for 1 to 2 minutes until soft and warmed through. Next, add the avocado cream sauce into the pan and stir until well combined.

- Plate the zoodles and top with chicken. Enjoy!

4. EGGVOCADO BOATS

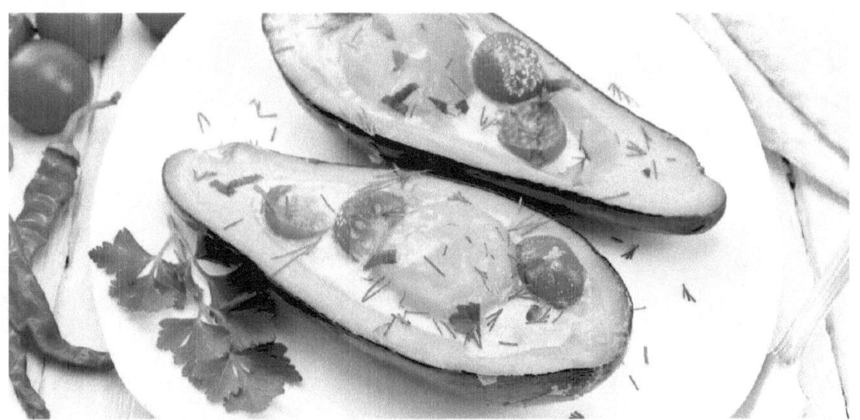

INGREDIENTS

- Cherry Tomatoes (halved) – ½ cup

- Fresh Dill (optional, to garnish) – ¼ tsp

- Sea Salt & Black Pepper (a pinch to taste) – 1/16 tsp

- Avocado – 1

- Eggs - 2

DIRECTIONS

- Preheat oven to 350°F (177°C).

- Slice the avocado in half and remove the pit. Scoop out a little flesh from each half to make room for the eggs. Place face-up on a baking sheet.

- Crack one egg in each half of the avocado. Bake for 10 to 15 minutes, depending on how runny you like your eggs.

- Take out of the oven and plate. Garnish with cherry tomatoes, scooped out avocado flesh, and fresh dill. Enjoy!

1. SALMON IN LEMON BUTTER SAUCE

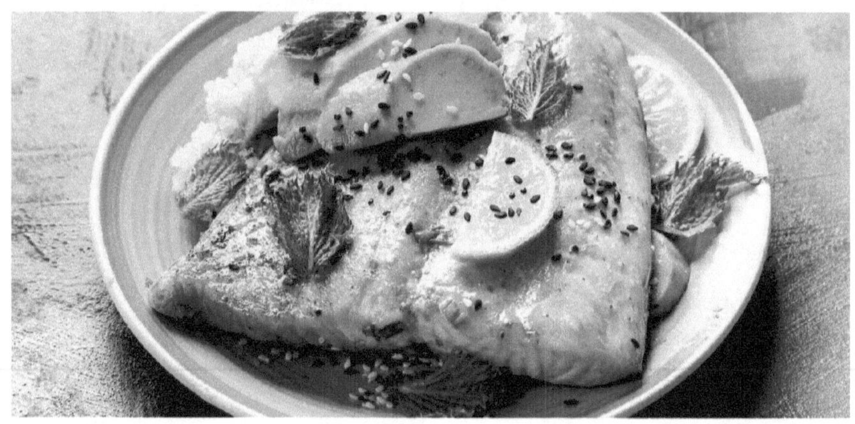

INGREDIENTS

- Avocado Oil – ½ tsp

- Salmon Fillet – 125 grams

- Garlic (cloves, minced) - 2

- Capers – 1 tbsp

- Lemon Juice – 1/4

- Butter – 1 tablespoon

- Avocado (Sliced) - 1/8

- Sesame Seeds (to sprinkle on top) - 1/8 tsp

DIRECTIONS

- Wash and dry the salmon.

- Heat the avocado oil in a pan over medium heat and add the salmon skin side up to the pan — Cook for 1 to 2 minutes. Then flip to the other side and cook for another minute.

- Remove the pan from the heat and cover with a lid for 5 to 10 minutes until the salmon is cooked through. Divide onto plates and cover to keep the salmon warm.

- Add the capers, garlic, and lemon juice to the same pan. Cook over medium heat for 3 minutes, then turn off the heat and stir in the butter until melted.

- Drizzle the capers and lemon butter sauce over the salmon. Add the avocado slices and sprinkle with sesame seeds. Enjoy!

2. KETO QUESADILLAS

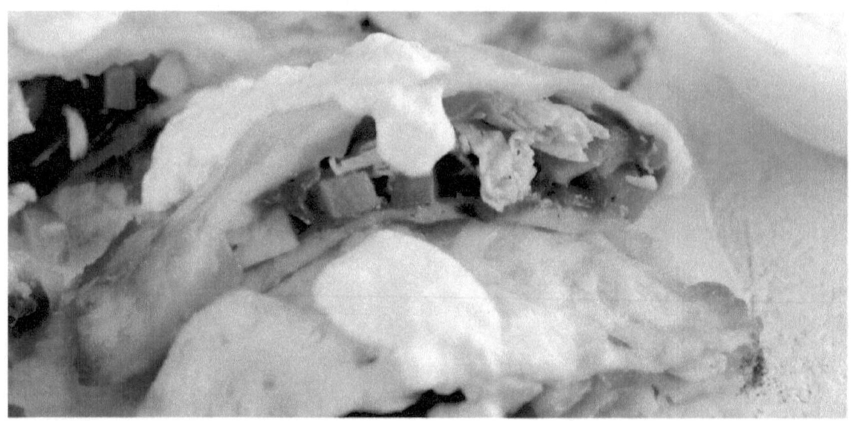

INGREDIENTS

- Sour Cream (for decoration) – 2 tbsp

- Green Onion (thinly sliced) – ½ stalk

- Avocado (thinly sliced) – ½

- Chicken Breast (shredded) – 60 grams

- Cheddar Cheese (Shredded) – 1 ¼ cup

- Monterey Jack (shredded) – 1 ¼ cup

- Sea Salt & Black Pepper (to taste) – 1/8 tsp

- Yellow Onion (sliced) - ¼

- Chili powder - ¼ tsp

- Red Bell Pepper (sliced) – ½

- Avocado Oil – 1 ½ tsp

DIRECTIONS

- Preheat oven to 400 °F.

- Line a medium baking sheet with parchment paper.

- Heat the avocado oil in a medium skillet over medium-high heat. Add the onions and red bell pepper and season with salt, pepper, and chili powder. Cook for 5 minutes until soft and transfer to a plate.

- Add the cheeses to a small bowl and mix well. Then take 1 1/2 cups of cheese mixture and add to the center of one of the prepared baking sheets. Spread the cheese mixture into an even layer in the shape of a circle in the size of a flour tortilla.

- Bake the cheese tortilla for 8 to 10 minutes until melty and slightly golden around the edge.

- Take out of the oven and add the shredded chicken, the onion-pepper mixture, and avocado slices to one half of the cheese tortilla. Let cool for a minute. With the help of a small spatula and the parchment paper, try to gently lift and fold the empty side of the cheese tortilla over the side with the fillings.

- Return to the oven and bake for another 3 to 4 minutes. In case you prepare more servings, repeat until you have used up all ingredients.

- Once done, cut the quesadilla into quarters. Divide onto plates and garnish with green onion and sour cream. Enjoy!

3. RAW VEGAN WALNUT TACOS

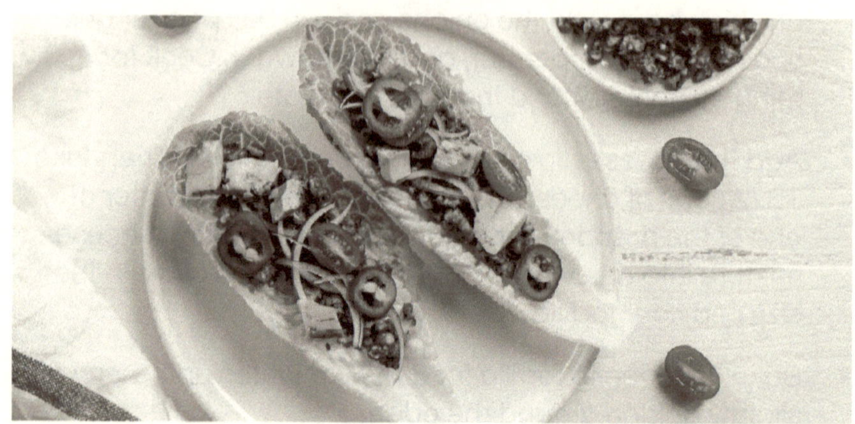

INGREDIENTS

- Cumin – 1 tsp

- Balsamic Vinegar – 1 ½ tsp

- Walnuts (raw) – ¾ cup

- Romaine Hearts (leaves separated, washed and dried) – 1/2

- Cherry Tomatoes (halved) – 1/3 cup

- Jalapeno Pepper (thinly sliced) - 1/2

- Red Onion (thinly sliced) – 2 tablespoons

- Avocado (cubed) – ½

- Garlic Powder – 1/16 tsp

- Chili Powder – 1/8 tsp

- Tamari – ¾ tsp

DIRECTIONS

- To the bowl of a food processor, add the walnuts, garlic, tamari, cumin, chili powder, and balsamic vinegar. Pulse a few times until well combined, and the walnuts are crumbly like ground meat.

- Add the ground mixture to romaine leaves and top with tomatoes, red onion, jalapeno, and avocado. Serve and enjoy!

NOTES

- Refrigerate the walnut taco mixture in an airtight container for up to two days.

- One serving is equal to approximately two romaine lettuce tacos.

4. ROASTED KETO CHICKEN WITH BROCCOLI AVOCADO AND GARLIC

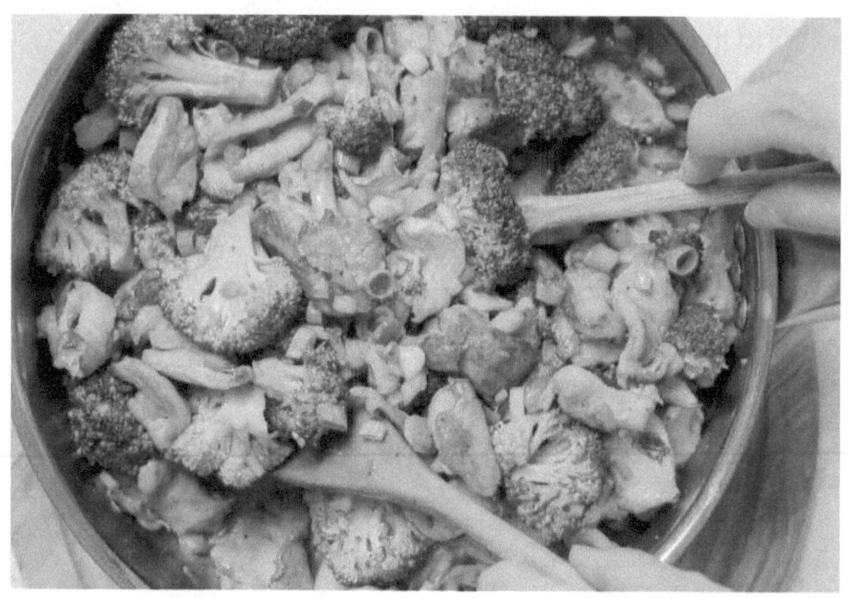

INGREDIENTS

- Oregano – 2 tbsps

- Garlic (cloves, peeled) - 3

- Sea Salt & Black Pepper – ½ tsp

- Broccoli (chopped) – 1 cup

- Cherry Tomatoes – 1 1/3 cup

- Avocado (cubed) – ½

- Avocado Oil – 2 2/3 tbsps

- Chicken Leg, Boneless With skin – 300 grams

DIRECTIONS

- Preheat the oven to 375°F (190°C).

- Add the chicken, garlic cloves, tomatoes, cubed avocado, and broccoli to a baking dish. Coat in avocado oil then season with salt, pepper, and oregano.

- Place in the oven and cook for about 50 minutes until golden brown and cooked through.

- Let cool slightly, then divide onto plates and enjoy!

1. KETO HOT CHOCOLATE

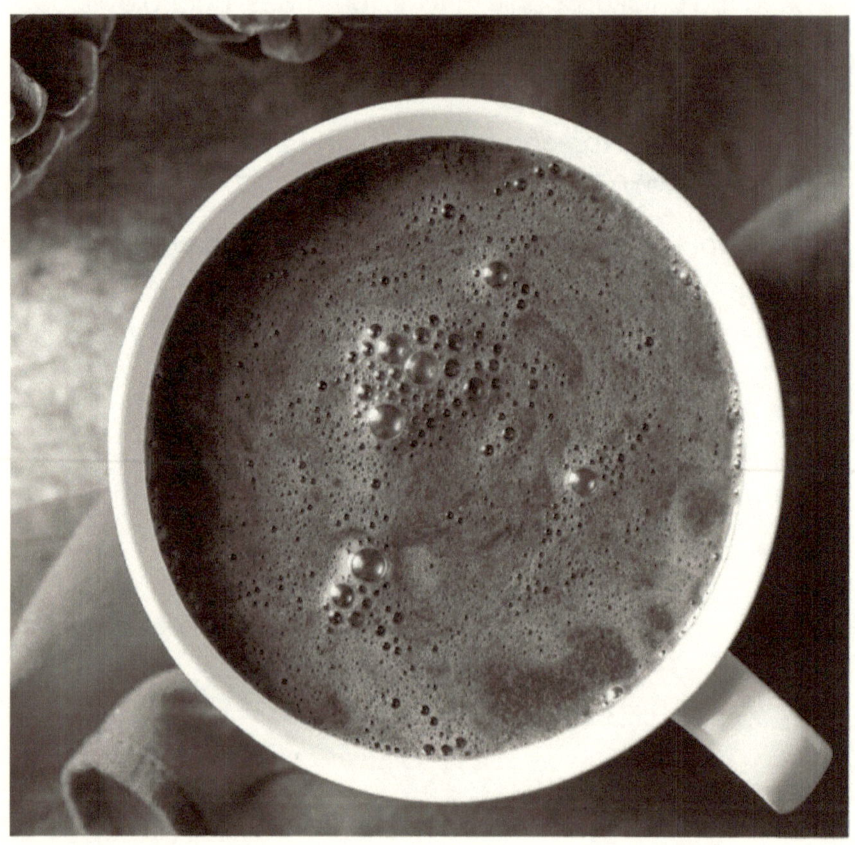

INGREDIENTS

- unsalted butter - 1 oz.

- Boiling water- 1 cup

- Powdered erythritol- 2½ tsp

- Vanilla extract - ¼ tsp

- Cocoa powder - 1 tbsp

DIRECTIONS

- Take a tall beaker, put all the ingredients and blend it until the texture changes into foam.

- Now, carefully pour the hot cocoa into the cups.

2. BULLET PROOF COFFEE

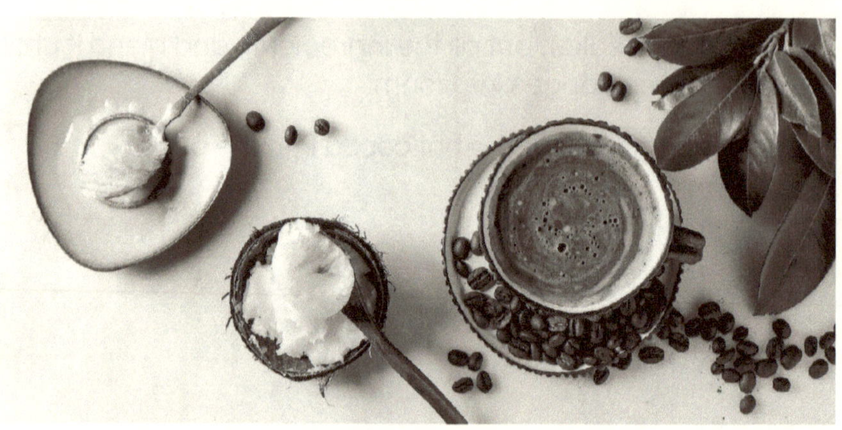

INGREDIENTS

- Organic Coffee (brewed) – 2 Cups

- MCT Coconut Oil- 1 tablespoon

- Butter (grass-fed butter) – 1 tablespoon

DIRECTIONS

- Brew or make your coffee as usual, using your preferred method. You will need around 2 cups of black coffee.

- Combine the butter and MCT oil in a blender.

- Pour the hot coffee over the butter and MCT oil and blend for a few seconds until smooth and frothy.

- Pour in a cup and enjoy

3. WHIPPED CREAM COFFEE

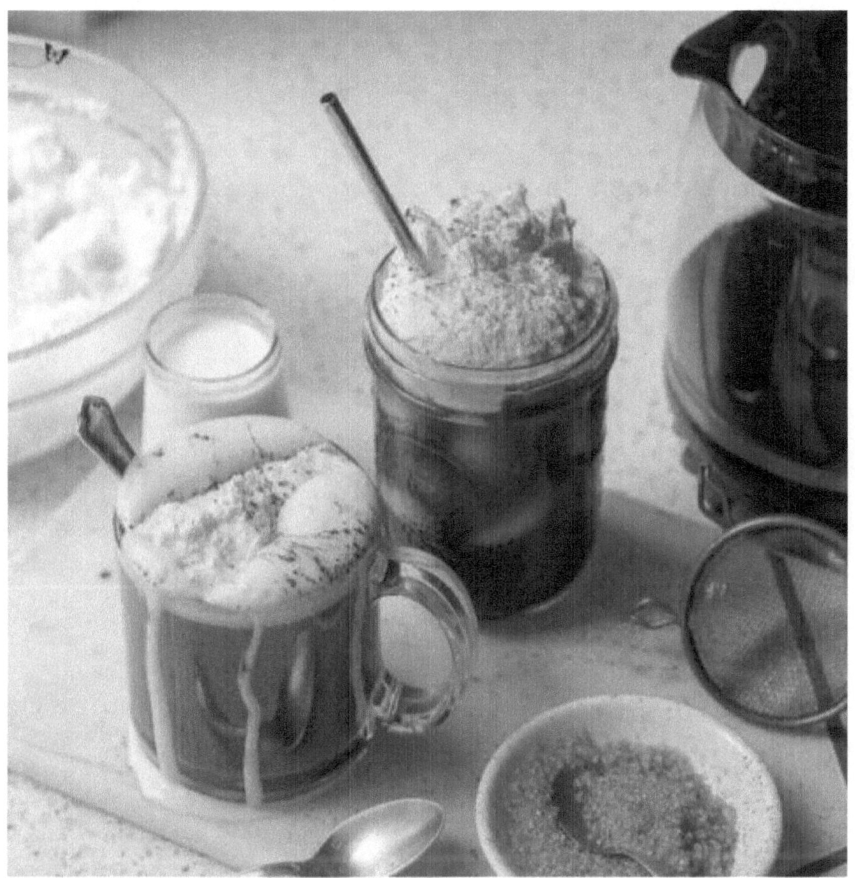

INGREDIENTS

- ground cinnamon or cocoa powder (optional)

- vanilla extract - ¼ tsp

- heavy whipping cream - ¼ cup

- coffee - 1 cup

DIRECTIONS

- Simply make coffee as you usually make it.

- Now take a bowl and add cream and vanilla extract in it and whip you see a foamy texture.

- Add coffee to a mug or a big cup. Pour the on top and sprinkle cinnamon or cocoa powder.

4. KETO GINGER SMOOTHIE

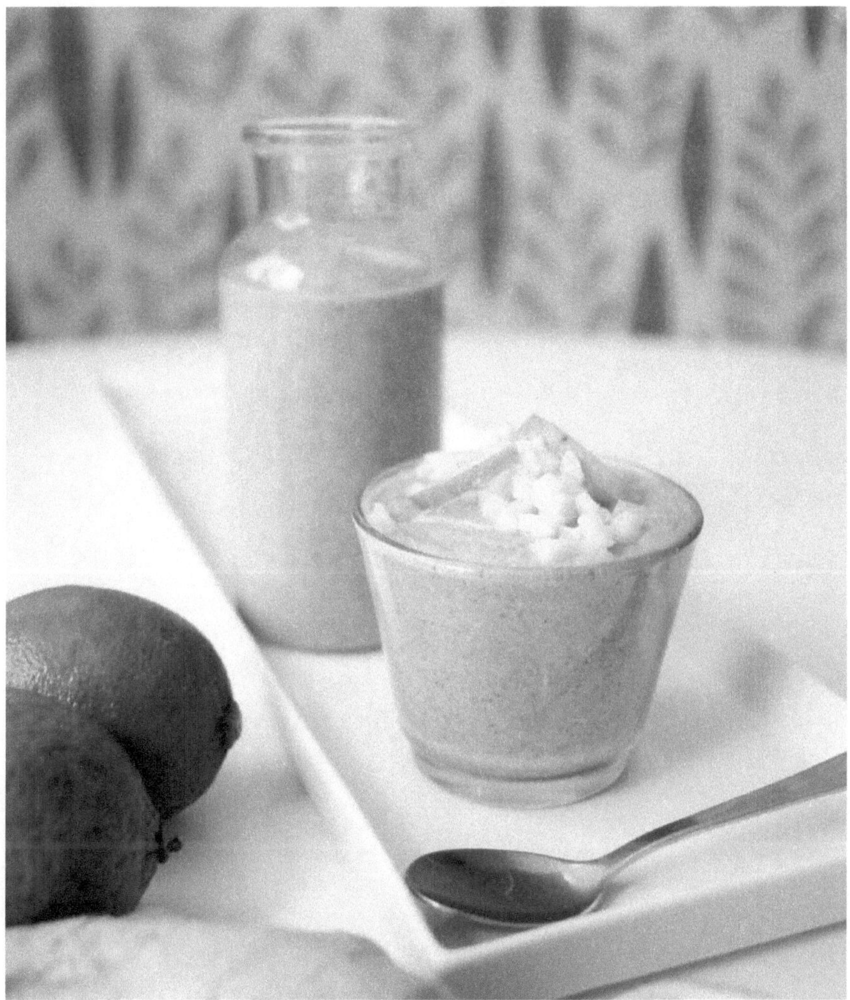

INGREDIENTS

- Fresh Ginger - 2 Tsp (Grated)

- Frozen Spinach - 1 Oz.

- Water - 2/3 Cup

- Coconut Cream Or Coconut Milk - 1/3 Cup

- Lime Juice - 2 Tbsp

DIRECTIONS

- You just need to mix all the above mentioned ingredients together.

- After this sprinkle it with grated ginger. Enjoy.

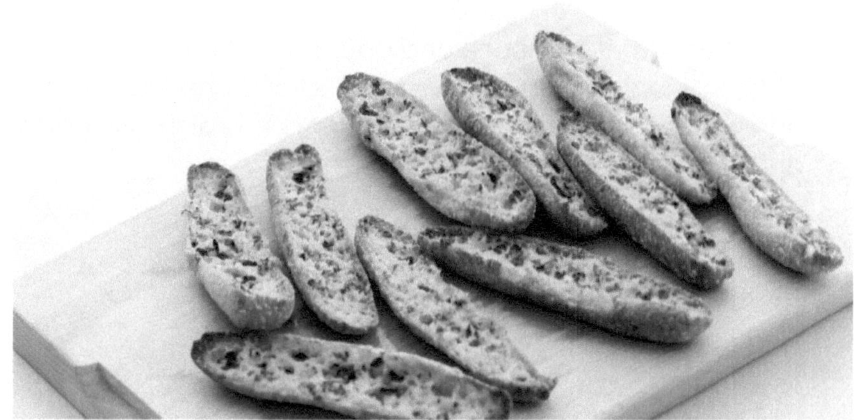

1. OVEN-BAKED KETO BRIE CHEESE

INGREDIENTS

- Pepper And Salt

- Camembert Cheese Or Brie Cheese - 9 Oz

- Fresh Rosemary - 1 Tbsp (Coarsely Chopped)

- Garlic Clove - 1 (Minced)

- Olive Oil - 1 Tbsp

- Walnuts Or Pecans - 2 Oz (Coarsely Chopped)

DIRECTIONS

- Simply preheat your oven to 200°C (400°F).

- Take a non-stick, small baking dish or a sheet pan and place the cheese on it.

- Mix the olive oil, nuts, herb and garlic together in a small bowl. Add pepper and salt to taste.

- Now take out the cheese and pour the nut mixture on it. After this, bake until nuts are roasted and cheese is soft and warm for about 10 minutes. Serve this dish lukewarm and warm.

2. KETO PANCAKES WHIPPED CREAM AND BERRIES

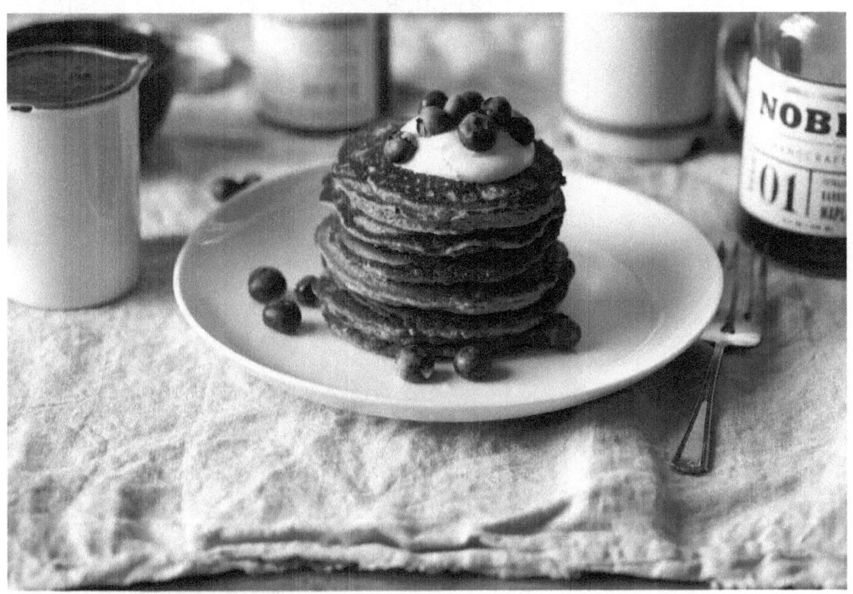

INGREDIENTS

For Pancakes

- Coconut Oil Or Butter - 2 Oz.

- Eggs- 4

- Psyllium Husk Powder - 1 Tbsp

- Cottage Cheese - 7 Oz.

Toppings For Pancakes

- Whipping Cream – 1 Cup and Fresh Strawberries Or Blueberries And Raspberries - 2 Oz.

DIRECTIONS

- Take a medium size bottle and add psyllium husk, cottage cheese and eggs and mix them. Let it rest for a few minutes. Now take a non-stick skillet and heat it up with oil and butter. On medium-low heat, fry the pancakes for 5 minutes.

- The next step is to take a separate bowl and add whip cream until it has a foamy texture. Use berries of your choice and whipped cream to serve with the pancakes.

3. HAZELNUT AND CHOCOLATE KETO SPREAD

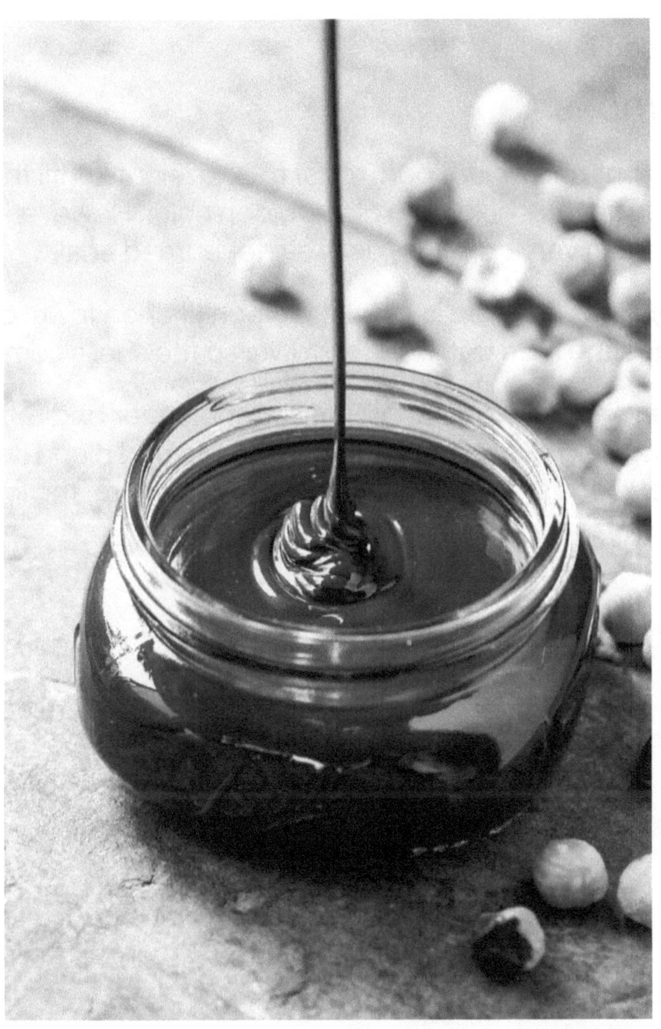

INGREDIENTS

- Erythritol - 1 Tsp (Optional)
- Hazelnuts - 5 Oz.

- Unsalted Butter - 1 Oz.

- Coconut Oil - ¼ Cup

- Vanilla Extract - 1 Tsp

- Cocoa Powder - 2 Tbsp

DIRECTIONS

- In a hot and dry fry pan, roast the hazelnuts until they change their color to a nice golden color. However, roast the nuts very carefully, as they get burned easily.

- Now the next step is to take a clean kitchen towel and place the nuts in it. Rub the towel so the shells come off.

- After this, take a food processor or blender and put the remaining ingredients along with nuts and blend it to desired consistency. The smoother the mixture, the longer you mix.

4. BUTTERCREAM IN KETO STYLE

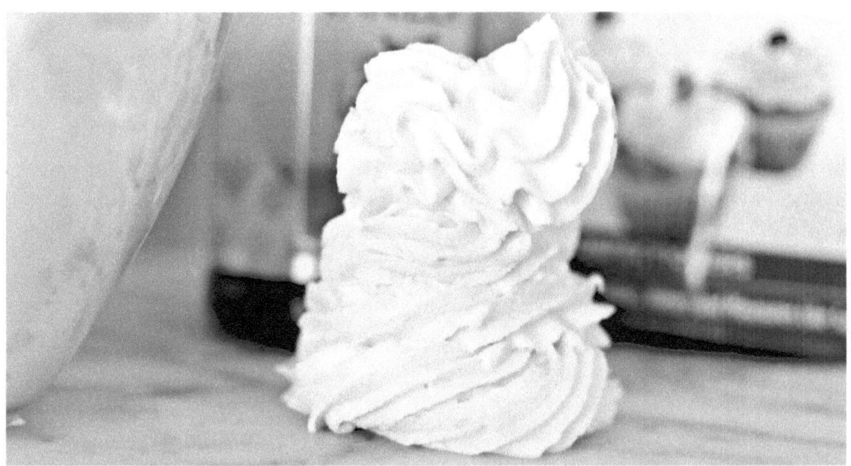

INGREDIENTS

- Erythritol - 1 Tsp (Optional)

- Unsalted Butter - 8 Oz. At Room Temperature

- Ground Cinnamon - 1½ Tsp

- Vanilla Extract - 2 Tsp

DIRECTIONS

- In a small pan, take ¼ of butter and heat it until it changes to amber in color. Make sure to not burn it.

- In a beaker, pour the browned butter and whisk in the remaining butter slowly using a hand mixer until it becomes fluffy.

- Finally, add optional sweetener, vanilla and cinnamon towards the end.

1. CELERY WITH ALMOND BUTTER

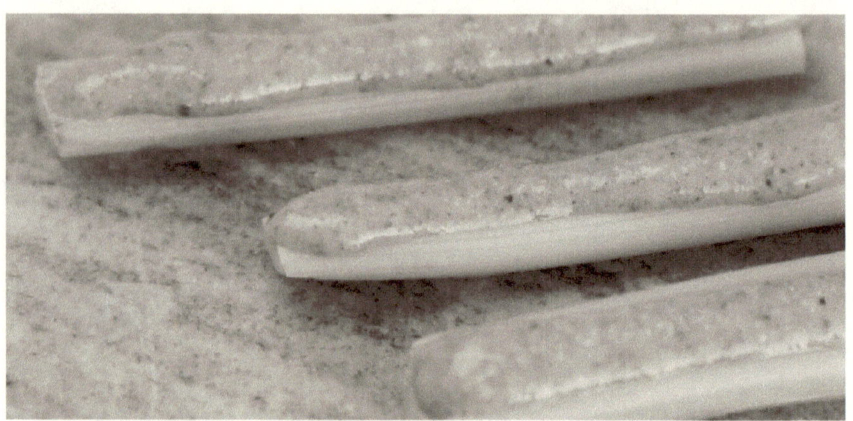

INGREDIENTS

- Celery (sliced into sticks) – 2 stalks

- Almond Butter – 2 tablespoons

DIRECTIONS

Spread almond butter across celery sticks (about 1 tbsp per celery stalk). Enjoy!

2. AVOCADO WEDGES WRAPPED IN SALMON

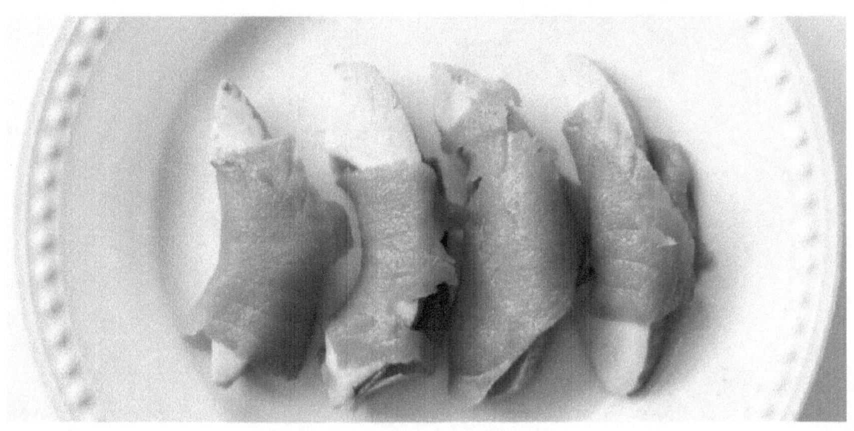

INGREDIENTS

- Avocado – 1/2

- Smoked Salmon (sliced) 50 grams

- Lemon (optional) – 1/4

DIRECTIONS

Slice the avocado into wedges and wrap each wedge with smoked salmon. Optionally drizzle fresh lemon juice on top. Plate and enjoy!

3. KETO EGGPLANT PIZZAS

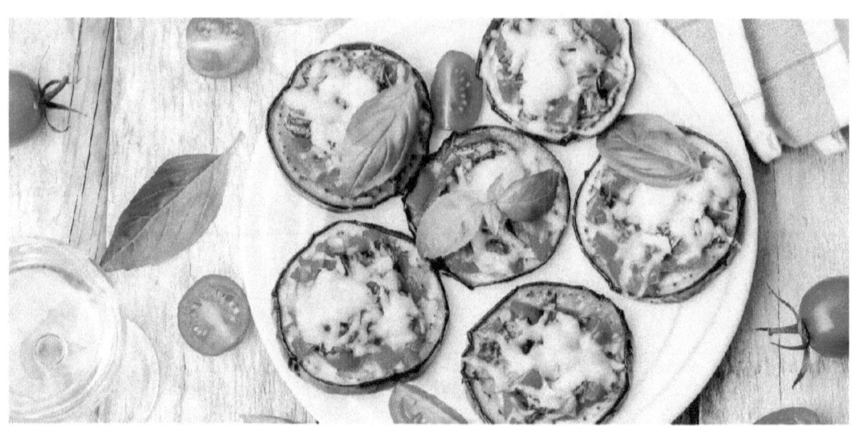

INGREDIENTS

- Eggplant (medium) – 1/2

- Extra Virgin Olive Oil – 2 tablespoon

- Himalayan Salt (to taste) - 1/8 tsp

- Black Pepper (to taste) - 1/8 tsp

- Tomato Sauce – 1/3 cup

- Oregano – ¼ tsp

- Mozzarella Ball (grated) – 63 grams

- Red Pepper Flakes (Optional) – ¼ tsp

- Basil Leaves (finely chopped) – 1 tablespoon

DIRECTIONS

- Cut the eggplant into 1/2 inch thick slices. Brush each side of the eggplant with oil and season with Himalaya salt and black pepper.

- Heat a non-stick pan over medium heat and cook the eggplant slices in batches for 3 to 5 minutes per side until tender and browned.

- While the eggplant slices are cooking, turn the broiler on high.

- Transfer the cooked eggplant slices to a baking sheet. Top each slice with the tomato sauce, sprinkle with dried oregano, and cover with some shredded cheese.

- Broil the 'eggplant pizzas' for 3 to 5 minutes until the cheese is melted and slightly browned.

- Remove from the oven and sprinkle with red pepper flakes and fresh basil. Plate and enjoy!

NOTES

Refrigerate in an airtight container for up to two days. Reheat in the oven until warmed through. One serving size is around 3 egg plants.

4. KETO FUDGE FAT BOMBS

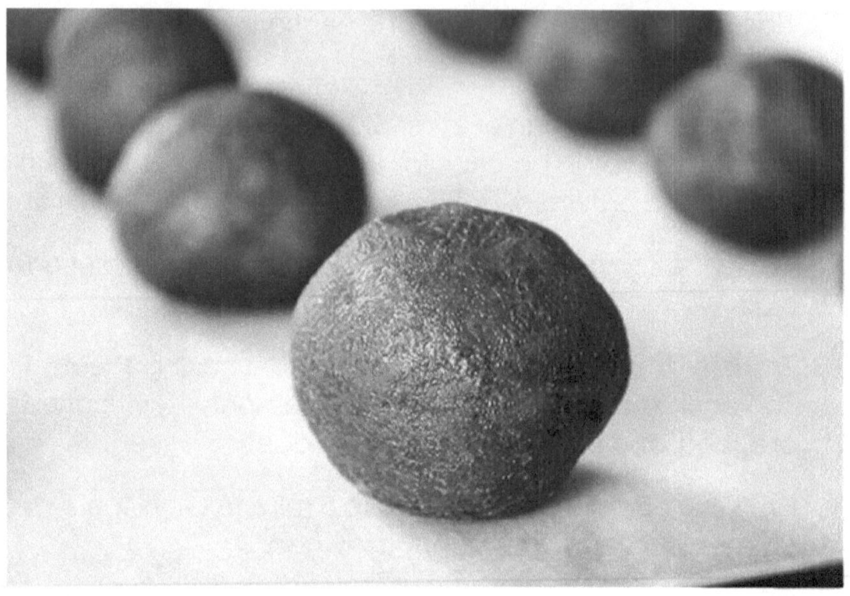

INGREDIENTS

- Almond Butter (no sugar added) – 2/3 cup

- Coconut Oil (liquid) – 2/3 cup

- Sea Salt (to taste) – 1/16 tsp

- Cocoa Powder (unsweetened) – 1/3 cup

- Stevia Powder – 1/3 tsp

- Coconut Flour – 3 1/8 tablespoon

DIRECTIONS

- Combine almond butter and coconut oil and in a small pot and melt over medium heat

- Add dried ingredients to the same pot and stir until well combined.

- Take off the heat and allow the mixture to cool slightly. Taste test a bit to determine if you need additional sweetener. Add more as necessary, depending on your liking.

- Pour the mixture into a bowl and transfer to your freezer to solidify for approximately 60-90 minutes.

- Once solidified, remove the bowl from your freezer and form the mixture into balls. Place the formed balls on a flat tray or plate and return to the freezer for 15-20 minutes. Enjoy! *Tip: To prevent the coconut oil from melting in your hands while forming the balls, wash your hands under cold water and wipe with a dry paper towel.

NOTES

- You can store your fat bombs in an airtight container in your freezer. Then, when you want one, simply pop one fat bomb out and let it thaw for a few minutes before eating it.

- Two Fat bombs equal one serving.

CONCLUSION

This ebook 'Fat Does Not Make You Fat' is a great treat for people looking to lose weight in a healthy way. Obesity has so many harmful effects for your body. If you are suffering from severe obesity, then chances to get different diseases become very high. Obesity impacts your body dramatically. The symptoms of obesity can be harmful to your physical and mental health. You may suffer from diabetes, heart diseases, joints and muscle problems because of obesity. To beat obesity, first you should know the root cause of obesity

High insulin levels, also known as hyperinsulinemia results in obesity. Fructose is another element that develops high levels of insulin. Overtime the continuous consumption of fructose results in higher levels of insulin, which lead to obesity. Some people try cutting their calories to lose weight. However, when you take calories less than your body needs, it makes you feel exhausted, and it becomes difficult for you to cover up with your daily nutrient requirements. For instance, low-calorie diets may cause deficiency of vitamin B12, folate or iron. Consequently, you may become anemic and experience extreme fatigue.

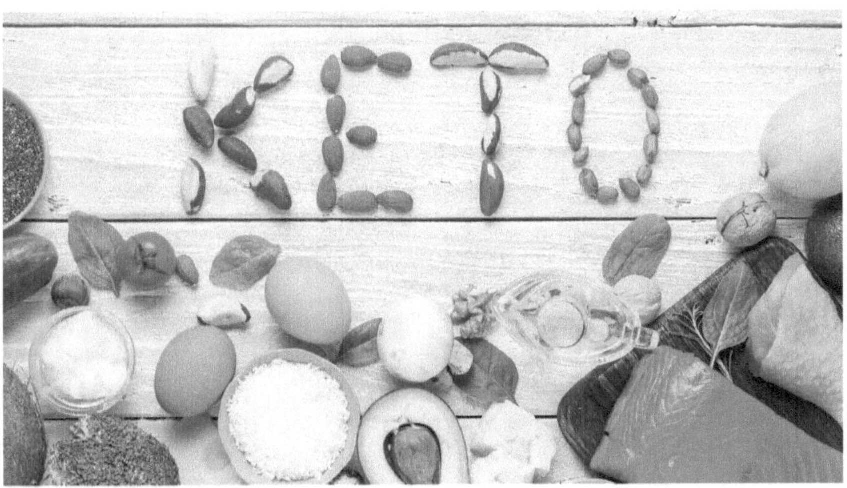

If you wish to lose pounds in less time period, low-carb diet, also known as keto diet is definitely a better solution. Its effectiveness increases, if you combine it with intermittent fasting. The low carb diet helps you in maintaining a normal eating schedule, at the same time, keeping insulin levels in range and lower storage of fat. When keto diet and fasting are done together, it provides health benefits, such as increased energy, increased focus, reduced blood pressure and cholesterol levels and weight loss.

The first step to changing your lifestyle is the fact that you have finally decided to try intermittent fasting and keto together. This clearly shows that you not only want to improve your health but also lose weight. The journey to have a successful keto diet becomes easier if you keep tracking your food and be consistent.

So what are you waiting for? Try the amazing keto diet along with intermittent fasting to keep yourself healthy and achieve your fitness goals now!